HONED

HONED

FINDING YOUR EDGE AS A MAN OVER 40

MIKE SIMPSON, MD

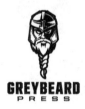

GREYBEARD
P R E S S

HONED

Finding Your Edge as a Man Over 40

ISBN   978-1-5445-2241-8 *Hardcover*

978-1-5445-2240-1 *Paperback*

978-1-5445-2239-5 *Ebook*

To my wife, Denise: you make it easy for me to stay young because my life didn't actually start until the day we met.

CONTENTS

INTRODUCTION

Two blacked-out Chinook helicopters cut their way through the night sky over northern Afghanistan. Inside the lead aircraft, I shifted in my seat to get some circulation back in my legs. As blood flow returned to my muscles and nerves, I once again felt the mechanical hum of the aircraft vibrating up through my feet.

"Two minutes!" came over my radio headset from the platoon leader.

We were two minutes out from the designated landing zone (LZ) where our mission would begin. Stepping on the scale before the mission, the total weight of my gear was just over 90 pounds. Shifting in my seat now I certainly felt it, but that was nothing compared to what I knew I would feel during the hours that lay ahead as the mission took me through the rugged Afghanistan mountains. I conducted a quick head-to-toe inspection to ensure that I had all my gear, and everything was secure. Helmet: check; night-vision goggles: check; radio: check; M4 carbine: check; pistol: check; medic bag: check. A final tug at my body armor and a trace of my fingers over the fully loaded carbine magazines across my chest, and I knew I was ready.

"One minute!"

All of us onboard slid out of our seats and took a knee facing the rear of the aircraft. I flipped my night-vision goggles (NVGs) down and did a quick scan around me through their green illumination. The 15 Rangers crowded around me did the same, all ensuring that none of our gear was accidentally left behind. Looking over my shoulder, I saw the Chinook crew chief hunch his shoulders, training his machine gun on the nearby ridge as we descended. The pitch of the rotors changed, and a frigid rush of air assaulted us from the open ramp. We unclipped our safety lines the moment we felt the bump of the wheels touching the ground and rushed down the ramp and out into the night, forming a semi-circle and each dropping to a knee. As the two aircraft lifted off behind us, their rotor blades directed an arctic blast against our backs, and snow swirled around us. It was December 2013.

As the helicopters flew into the distance with the sound of the rotors receding with them, the deep quiet of the Afghan night settled around us. Without a word, we rose as one and turned to move off of the LZ. The icy crunch as our boots penetrated the top layer of snow was all that anyone would hear. What lay ahead of us was an eight-kilometer movement through some of the most difficult terrain in northern Afghanistan, ultimately to arrive at our objective: a remote village that was home to at least four high-level Taliban insurgents.

As we moved off the LZ and started our route northward, the platoon sergeant counted each member of the platoon to ensure that no one had been left behind on the aircraft or the LZ. I was towards the back of the formation, and he recognized me as I passed, giving me a squeeze on my shoulder. Other than me, he was the oldest person on this mission. This was the 29th year of my service in uniform, and many of the Rangers on this patrol had not even been born when I first raised my right hand and took the oath of enlistment back in 1984. This was certainly something I had reflected upon leading up to the mission. Just the day before, I had made the comment that, at 48 years old, I was the same age my father had been when I started my military career with the Rangers. I pondered for a moment how the younger version of me would have viewed going on a combat patrol with a man my father's age. Certainly, my participation in this mission was an outlier. Not only was I older than anyone else in the group, but I was also a board-certified emergency medicine physician. It's certainly not what most people would expect when they think about a platoon of Rangers on a combat mission to engage the Taliban. Just as my presence on this mission could be considered somewhat atypical, so was the journey through life that had led me to this moment.

In June of 1984, just two weeks out of high school, I shipped off to basic training at Fort Benning, Georgia. That would begin my first four-year enlistment as an infantryman in the First Ranger Battalion. Life as an Airborne Ranger was everything I had imagined it would be. Each day was a challenge. Some days were more difficult for me than for my fellow Rangers. At only 5′6″, I was shorter than most of my peers, and many of the physical tasks were slightly more difficult for me. My legs were shorter, which meant keeping up on runs was more difficult. Things like obstacle courses and performing tasks in full gear were often times more challenging. A "combat load" that was less than a third of a larger peer's body weight was nearly 50 percent of mine. Although all of this made for some interesting physical challenges, I never let any of it get in my way. I never allowed myself to be the weakest link, and I always kept up with my squad in everything we did. And when I was promoted to sergeant, I led from the front. Always.

I encountered similar challenges when I transitioned to

a career in Special Forces, first as an engineer sergeant and, ultimately, as a Special Forces medic. Even though the physical tasks never came as easily to me as they did to my more genetically gifted peers, I always maintained the standard in all that I did—even if that meant putting in a little extra work to stay physically fit.

Ultimately, after what most would consider to be an extremely successful 17-year career as an operator, I left that life to accept an officer's commission and attend medical school, eventually becoming an emergency medicine physician. My goal from the very beginning was to return to special operations and to provide the best medical care possible to those who serve at the tip of the spear. I was fortunate in achieving that goal with a coveted assignment to the Joint Medical Augmentation Unit (JMAU) under the Joint Special Operations Command (JSOC) at Fort Bragg, North Carolina. The JMAU is highly unique in that it is the only Tier 1 special operations medical unit providing direct medical support to JSOC special mission units. It was because of my assignment to the JMAU that I was afforded the privilege to walk a combat patrol with the very same Ranger Battalion I had been assigned to in the 1980s. But even though my assignment had gotten me there, I knew I had to prove myself. I knew I had to prove to the Rangers that I was an asset on the battlefield and not a liability (for to be a liability meant that, at best, I would be left behind on future missions, and at worst, I could be the cause of mission failure).

At age 48, keeping up with operators less than half my age was no small feat, and just a few years before, I would not have thought it possible. Because of my nontraditional journey, I graduated medical school at age 40. The rigors of internship, including long shifts, little time off, and 24-hour call rotations, all took a much greater toll on my body than they did on my younger classmates. By the time I was assigned to the JMAU, I was already facing the physical challenges of middle age in my mid-40s. At a time when most men my age were shifting down into second gear to relax and look back on their accomplishments, I was shifting into high gear and preparing to deploy in the Global War on Terror (GWOT) with the most elite units in the United States military. Looking in the mirror, stepping on the scale, and struggling with workouts in the gym all validated my growing concern: I had lost what career soldiers refer to as "the edge." Just as the blade of a sword may lose sharpness over time, an old soldier can also lose his ability to perform at peak physical level as he ages. The sharp "edge" that I had diligently maintained in my younger years was now gone, but I was determined to get it back.

Through trial and error, I discovered that the approach to physical fitness and mission readiness that had served me as an operator in my 20s and 30s was not sufficient to prepare or sustain me in my 40s. Utilizing my medical training, I sought out every book I could get my hands on and consulted with every expert I could find on what I needed

to do to keep up with the operator lifestyle. Fitness, nutrition, supplementation—I researched it all. On that winter
night in the mountains of Afghanistan, on my fifth and final
combat deployment with the JMAU, I was able to really see
how my hard work paid off and what kind of shape I was
really in. This was a "final exam" of sorts.

As we neared the objective, I felt great. There was never a
moment where I had fallen behind or where I had failed to
maintain security and a tactical bearing during the movement. The brisk movement over the steep and rugged
Afghan terrain had certainly been strenuous, and the sweat,
running out from under my helmet and down my face, now
formed ice crystals on my thick deployment beard. I looked
forward to a brief rest at the rally point near the objective,
which would be an opportunity to take a knee and drink
some water while the command element went forward to
conduct a reconnaissance.

As we spread out to move across a small open area just prior
to the rally point, the distinct sound of AK-47 fire rang out
from the high ground above us. Together, like one creature,
we broke into a run across the uneven terrain toward the
cover of thick brush on the ridge line, which flanked the
objective. Not slowing down as we hit the concealment
of the vegetation, we moved in a bounding formation up
the ridge, slowing just shy of the crest. A low rock wall ran
along the top of the ridgeline, paralleling the buildings,

which comprised our designated objective. Just as we have been trained, we took up positions along the wall equally spaced, hunkered down low, our weapons trained on the buildings where the gunfire had come from. To my left and right, I could hear the ragged breathing of the Rangers in the squad around me, some breathing harder than others. For a moment, I took stock of my own breathing and heart rate and did a quick self-assessment. Even after a long and difficult movement, even after a surge of adrenaline and an uphill sprint in full combat gear, I was far from played out. As I caught my breath, I felt very confident that I had plenty of gas left in the tank. There in the darkness, atop that ridge in Afghanistan, I smiled to myself. Even at age 48, I still had "the edge" and could still function as an operator. I was still in the fight.

In the years that passed since that night in Afghanistan, I have continued to push myself physically and have expanded my knowledge as it applies to keeping that "edge" as I grow older. In 2016, when I was given my retirement physical in preparation to separate from the military, I finally appreciated the true toll that the years of service had taken on my body. The multiple MRIs and physical exams exposed every injury that I had chosen to ignore over the course of my career.

The reality of the situation was that I was now a 50-year-old former operator with an extensive list of injuries. But, rather than allowing that reality to become an excuse to lead a sedentary lifestyle, I chose to instead increase my focus on both physical fitness and the practice of martial arts. I continued to conduct my own research on all topics related to health and fitness, to consult with colleagues and reach out to experts, and I made it a point to share everything I learned on my podcast "Mind of The Warrior." It was because of the exposure provided by the podcast that I frequently found myself being asked for advice, usually from men who were right around my age and were facing similar challenges. I began to notice a distinct pattern in the questions—about exercise, nutrition, sleep, supplements, mindset, and all of the things that I had wrestled with and studied on my own. Eventually, it dawned on me that, although my story was unique to me, the lessons I was learning and the questions they answered were fairly common among like-minded men in my age group.

At this point, you may be asking yourself if this book is right for you, so allow me to lay out specifically who I had in mind when I set out to write it.

Bottom line: if you are a man who is over 40 and wants more in the way of health, fitness, and quality of life, then this book is written especially for you. Based upon my experience and observations, the men who are likely to want and need the information contained in this book tend to fall into four categories: those who were in great shape in their younger years but have now allowed fitness to become low priority, those who have continued to work out but who now feel it is more of a struggle, those who may have been sidelined by injuries, and what I call the "late bloomers" who haven't previously put a lot of effort into their fitness but have decided that it is time for a lifestyle change.

I have gotten many emails from men who were once high school/collegiate athletes or possibly served a few years in the military in their younger years. They talk about looking back on those years and longing to feel that way again, but they don't know how to get there. If you fall into this category, this book will help you recapture the feeling of health and vigor that you knew in your youth through an understanding of what constitutes a truly healthy lifestyle, not just in the area of fitness and nutrition, but also in recovery, sleep, and attitude.

For those who have continued to work out as they age, many reach a point where they feel like they just aren't getting the results that they used to. They may be experiencing a feeling similar to walking up a hill that seems to become progressively steeper as the years pass. Also, they may feel that whatever it is they are doing in their workout routine doesn't seem to translate into a better lifestyle. If this describes you, this book will help you understand the effects of aging and why the workout routine that you have done for years may no longer be suitable to keep you in shape. It will also help you to determine what your fitness goals are and how to structure all aspects of your lifestyle to reach them.

As injuries are something I have dealt with myself, I am acutely aware of the challenges that they can present when it comes to achieving and maintaining a high level of fitness. If you are like me in this regard, then this book will help you better understand how to structure a workout that will help you strengthen your weak areas and diminish the aggravation of your injuries. Through a well-rounded program, proper rest, and natural supplementation, you will be able to navigate your way to a life of health and optimal performance in spite of your battle scars.

Those that fall into the "late bloomer" category typically use language like, "I have always wanted to____, but____," or they ask questions like, "Is it too late for me to start_____ at my age?" My response is that if you want something bad enough, then you just do it, and the only time that it's too late to start *anything* is when you are dead. If this sounds like you, then the time is now, and this book is for you. This book will provide you the starting point that you need, and a road map on how to reach your ultimate destination once you determine what that happens to be. By gaining scientifically sound and easy-to-follow principles on all aspects of a healthy lifestyle, you will realize that the years ahead of you can be the best of your life as long as you are willing to take that first step.

You may fall into one of these categories, or you may see a bit of yourself in more than one. Or you may just be an "average" man who has reached his 40th year on earth, and you want to strive to be above average. However you happen to define yourself, let me be your guide in how you rewrite your story going forward and *redefine* yourself as what I like to call a *warrior-athlete*. If that catches your interest, then take the first step with me, and turn the page as I define exactly what that means and how we get there, together.

CHAPTER 1

PERFORMANCE VS. LONGEVITY FOR THE WARRIOR-ATHLETE

In June of 1984, I walked out the front door of my parents' home in California and got into a car with the Army recruiter who drove me to the processing center to enter the United States Army. Had you asked me that day if I was embarking on a journey to live life as a warrior, I would have said, "Yes," but I honestly didn't really know at the time what that meant. The life of a warrior isn't just about being proficient in weapons and tactics, nor is it as simple as being physically fit, although all of those things play a part.

The word "warrior" gets thrown around a lot in this day and age. Much like the word "hero," the word "warrior" has come to mean virtually anyone working towards a goal. The flip side of the coin is that some people have attached negative connotations to the word "warrior," seemingly lumping it into the same category as "war monger." When the United States Army initiated a new public relations campaign that involved referring to soldiers as "warriors," a certain segment of over-sensitive and under-educated staff officers launched a movement aimed at convincing the Army to abandon the term. They stated (incorrectly) that warriors were the equivalent of mercenaries, who lacked the discipline and adaptability of soldiers. Bullshit. (To be fair, they were correct in stating that *not all* soldiers are warriors. In truth, only around ten percent of the military can be considered warriors.) Around the same time, certain local municipalities throughout the U.S. sought to ban law enforcement officers from attending what was referred to as "warrior training," which some government bureaucrats naively postulated might cause police officers to act as if the neighborhoods where they worked were war zones filled with bloodthirsty terrorists. Again: bullshit.

What neither the politicians nor the staff officers understood is what it is that truly makes someone a warrior. In simple terms, a warrior is someone who lives by a code. This code has come to be known as *the warrior ethos*. A warrior is selfless and places the safety of others over his own personal well-being. Likewise, he places the success of *the mission* over his own needs and comforts as an individual. A warrior is honorable and protects the weak. Most importantly, a warrior dedicates himself to becoming the best possible version of himself that he can be and does not shirk from the difficult tasks involved in the realization of that goal. A warrior does not make excuses, and he doesn't quit when things become difficult. *That* is the mentality of a warrior.

You may be thinking that the term "warrior" doesn't apply to you, but I believe it does. Allow me to illustrate.

If you approach health and fitness as a "hobby" or as a "chore" then you will never be 100 percent committed to the task. But if you approach it as a warrior, dedicating yourself to putting in the hard work required to maximize your physical fitness, you will be able make it the centerpiece of your lifestyle. By embracing the warrior ethos and placing the mission of optimal health and wellness ahead of other pursuits, you can unlock your life as a *warrior-athlete*.

Just as a warrior keeps his weapon, his equipment, and his body in battle-ready condition at all times, so a warrior-athlete places supreme importance on every aspect of his physical fitness. To be a warrior-athlete means leaving all excuses behind and realizing that your health and wellness are *your* responsibility and yours alone. It means leading a life of continued self-improvement, striving to be the best possible version of yourself that you can be, not just for today, but for a lifetime.

As someone who dedicated himself to being a warrior at a young age and now looks back as a "Greybeard," I am acutely aware of some of the pitfalls I encountered along the way. The focus of this chapter (and, indeed, of this book as a whole) is to help illustrate those pitfalls so that you may avoid them on your journey as a warrior-athlete.

In 2016, I retired from the United States Army with 32 years of active service. Half of that time, the first half, had been spent as an operator in Special Operations Forces (SOF). Largely because of how I lived my life during that first half of my career, I received a 100 percent disability classification from the Veterans Administration (VA) upon my retirement. Missing cartilage and torn ligaments in both knees, an unhealed 30-year-old fracture in my left foot, four herniated discs in my spine, two bad shoulders, and numerous other chronic injuries—these internal scars serve as testimony to the manner in which I sacrificed my body at the altar of mission readiness. As I stated earlier, the mission is everything, and accomplishing the mission is paramount, even at the expense of personal injury.

When I began my military career in the 1980s, physical fitness was very much geared toward short-term mission accomplishment at the expense of the long-term health and longevity of the individual soldier. Indeed, soldiers were, in fact, looked upon as expendable commodities. As harsh as that sounds, it was true and still is to some extent. The main focus during that period was on the ability of the unit and the individual to conduct the mission at hand *right now*. No consideration was given to the long-term effects of a fast-paced and extremely intense training regimen over time. The result was that many soldiers of that era would be combat ineffective by their late 30s. This was a byproduct of a focus on performance optimization for the short term and was compounded by the fact that there was very little applied science as it related to physical fitness. This problem was not limited to the military but was also prevalent in professional sports of the era. This was a time when professional sports teams would conduct "no water" practices in the hope that they could condition players to perform efficiently with less hydration. Although techniques such as this seem ludicrous in retrospect, they were not at all uncommon at the time. From the level of the high school gym teacher up to the most elite military unit and professional sports team, most of what was done in the name of physical conditioning and strength training was based on tradition and anecdotal evidence as opposed to scientific data. Even though the application of science in the field of functional fitness has greatly advanced over recent decades, a common pitfall that still prevails is the focus on performance optimization at the expense of longevity optimization. Allow me to explain.

The term *performance optimization* refers to training with the focus of maximizing athletic performance in the short term. Probably the most classic example of this would be a professional fighter undergoing a "fight camp" in the lead up to a professional bout. Militarily, this is best demonstrated in the form of a pre-deployment/pre-mission training cycle. Regardless of whether we are referring to a professional sports contest or a military operation, the goal is the same: conduct training that is as intense and realistic as humanly possible, with the goal of "peaking" in a narrow time window, which corresponds with the event in question. Anyone who has ever trained for any type of athletic competition is familiar with terms that coaches and trainers use, such as "ramping up." Although this training method may reap dividends on the playing field and even on the battlefield, it extracts a heavy toll from the warrior-athletes themselves. There's an old saying—"pay now, or pay later"—and certainly many of us know what it is like to "pay later."

When we are young, we feel that we are invincible. Injuries do not slow us down as much, and recovery times are much shorter. Our bones, joints, and soft tissues are much more forgiving of the mistakes we make and the punishment that we inflict upon them. This is essentially like living life on a credit card. A credit card with an extremely high limit and very low monthly payments but with an interest rate that compounds annually and continues to grow. By the time we reach middle-age, we will have amassed a crushing debt that is impossible to get out from under, if we have been continually living off of this "credit card."

In our youth, there is always that tendency to want to train just a little bit harder. We are constantly focused on short-term goals: the mission, the competition, losing the weight, getting in shape for the summer, or whatever it might be. Because we are not thinking about the future and are blinded to the long-term effects of our behavior, we often take shortcuts, and we often push too hard.

When I was in the Ranger Battalion, we were preparing for an upcoming training deployment, which I knew would entail a lot of long-range movement while carrying a heavy combat load. To better prepare myself and the Rangers under my supervision, I increased the days per week that we conducted road marches as a form of physical training. Additionally, I added extra weight to my own rucksack so that I would be better conditioned to carrying heavy loads. It was during that training that I started to notice a persistent pain in my left foot, especially when road marching on hard pavement. Years later, I discovered that I had caused a stress fracture in a bone and that, because I continued to walk on it without seeking medical attention, it never got a chance to heal. This was also the period of time when I started to notice numbness in my left arm any time I would wear my rucksack for an extended period. It wasn't until my retirement physical that I discovered I had permanent nerve damage in my arm, likely secondary to the amount of time I spent wearing a heavy rucksack. Unfortunately, sacrificing my body on the altar of performance optimization was not limited to my younger years. (In other words, I am a slow learner.) On a training cycle leading up to my deployment to Iraq in 2010, I spent extended periods of time wearing my Kevlar helmet with night vision goggles attached during nighttime training iterations. This was necessary, not only to get me accustomed to the added weight but also to help me overcome the claustrophobia and lack of depth perception while performing intricate tasks under NVGs. When I initially started to feel neck pain, I attributed it to muscle soreness from the weight of the helmet and NVGs. It wasn't until I got an MRI a few years later that I discovered I had actually herniated two of the discs in my cervical spine.

Indeed, virtually all of my chronic injuries can be traced to periods during my career when I tried to push just a little bit harder, when I tried to take shortcuts and ignored the pain signals my body was sending to me. In all of these instances, I was focused on the mission. I was focused on being ready "right now" and not concerned about any of the long-term effects that my extremely rigorous training might cause.

However, the damage inflicted in the name of performance optimization isn't limited to musculoskeletal injuries. Pushing too hard can mean damage due to secondary factors (such as severe dehydration, heat stroke, etc.) and can result in permanent damage to vital organs. The focus on performance optimization can cause someone to give in to the temptation to use performance-enhancing drugs. Do not be confused; that term isn't limited to substances such as steroids but can also mean the abuse or misuse of stimulants such as caffeine or nicotine to stay awake longer, train harder, and move farther faster. Addiction/ dependence on caffeine and nicotine is widespread in the military and can often be traced to the first few years of a soldier's initial enlistment. It was during Ranger school that I myself became dependent on chewing tobacco to stay awake and alert during periods of sleep deprivation. What started out as a "crutch" to keep from falling asleep ultimately became a 14-year habit that was extremely hard to break and damaged my gums to the point of requiring oral surgery. I was fortunate to not develop mouth cancer or any other serious long-term effects of my habit. Later, during my residency training as a new physician, I became dependent on energy drinks to keep going during long shifts. I developed headaches and discovered that my blood pressure was frighteningly high. I came dangerously close to having a stroke or doing permanent damage that could have adversely affected me for my entire life.

Both high-performance athletes and military operators also have trouble sleeping. In the case of athletes, it can be caused by over training and diet, as well as stimulant use in the form of caffeine or pre-workout formulas. For operators, it is due to multiple factors, compounded by the fact that most tactical missions are conducted at night, meaning that the mission sleep cycle occurs during the day. As inadequate sleep can become an impediment of performance optimization, those who have difficulty sleeping will often seek out ways to improve their situation. Bodybuilders have been known to resort to extreme measures, such as taking the drug gamma-hydroxybutyrate (GHB), which has been linked to long-term cognitive damage. Although not as extreme as GHB, the military community has a high degree of prescription sleep aid use. These medications are also not without risk of long-term problems. On a personal level, I have an extensive history of sleep difficulty, and during my operational years often had to utilize prescription sleep aids to get enough sleep to maintain mission readiness.

As you can see, many of the characteristics of performance optimization involve "running the engine in the red." Although this can certainly get you there fast and keep you in the race, it is unsustainable for indefinite periods and ultimately can lead to breakdown and disaster. Unfortunately, it sometimes is a necessary evil. One could ask, "How can you attain your long-term goals if you don't set short-term goals to get you there?" In spite of the impression that I may have given you, I am not saying that performance optimization is something to be shunned or avoided. On the contrary, performance optimization is something that you should strive for, but you should seek to do so intelligently and with minimal long-term cost. Remember, as a warrior-athlete, your health is the most important weapon in your arsenal, and you want to maintain it not just for the battle of today, but for every battle yet to come.

The flip side of the performance optimization coin is longevity optimization. *Longevity optimization* focuses on what is needed holistically to maintain the best overall health and fitness well past what would be considered the warrior-athlete's "prime." Optimizing longevity means recognizing that life is a marathon, not a sprint. Optimizing longevity means avoiding injury and not sacrificing long-term health for the sake of short-term goals. It means maintaining mission readiness at an acceptable level, if not a peak level, then for extended periods. Think of it as the reliable automobile that you drive for years as opposed to the sports car that you "run in the red" until it breaks down. This doesn't mean that optimizing longevity comes only at the exclusion of optimizing performance. On the contrary, the two can and do go hand in hand. Here's how.

NUMBER 1: THE WISDOM OF AGE

In decades past, both collectively and as individuals, we did not know what we did not know. Wisdom comes with age on both a personal level and in the broader sense. Simply put: we know quite a bit more today about fitness and injury prevention than we did 20 or 30 years ago. It is vitally important that you put this wisdom to use. Unlike the days of your youth, you now recognize that you are not invincible, and you have a much greater understanding of where your limits lie. It is because of these limits that you know exactly how far you can reasonably push yourself. This includes having an accurate assessment of your current state of fitness as well as a grasp on whatever injuries (both chronic and acute) that could possibly hinder your performance. Whatever method you choose in your approach to physical fitness and performance, optimization must be framed with this knowledge in mind. Remember, you no longer have the luxury of youth and its seemingly limitless healing powers. Be aware of your own mortality!

NUMBER 2: IT'S A MARATHON, NOT A SPRINT

The path to injury is paved with shortcuts. Too often, we concentrate on the short-term goals. This could mean an upcoming mission, a martial arts tournament that is just a few weeks away, or a triathlon or a 10K run that you delayed getting ready for. Remember, the key to results is consistency over time, not bursts of overly intense training on the quest to rapidly reach fitness goals. Too often, especially when we are trying to get back in shape after periods of inactivity, we expect results far too quickly. We allow ourselves to get discouraged when a week or two has passed and we do not feel any more fit, or the needle on the scale has not moved significantly. But you have to ask yourself, *Did I get out of shape in a week? Or was it over the period of months or years?* Personally, I had to come to grips with the fact that I could no longer get back into shape with two weeks of extremely intense exercise as I had done so many times in my younger years. Indeed, my middle-aged body is no longer capable of that. However long you spent getting out of shape, it will take you *at least* that long to get back into shape (and likely 30–50 percent longer).

Think of your personal fitness as points on a graph. If you were to engage in periods of high-intensity exercise and peak performance followed by periods of complete inactivity, the plot on that graph would look like a sawtooth pattern with "peaks and valleys." (Some of the "valleys" on the graph would likely be secondary to training injuries from pushing too hard.) On the other hand, if you maintained a consistent exercise program over time with the goal of achieving steady, incremental improvements, you would see a virtually straight line with an upward trajectory over the course of months and years with occasional plateaus. That is how you should envision your approach to physical fitness. Seek to be dedicated and consistent without concern for where you're going to be next week and more focus on where you're going to be five to ten years from now. That isn't to say that you may not occasionally ratchet up your intensity; certainly, you should. I always try to put in a "little extra" in my last workout right before a long weekend or business trip and have even been known to change gears in the weeks before I compete in Brazilian Jiu Jitsu. These are good practices as long as you execute them smartly. Simply put: do not allow yourself to be lured into "sprinting" towards short-term goals with reckless abandon at the expense of keeping up a steady jog that should last a lifetime.

NUMBER 3: HAVE A PLAN

Gone are the days when you can simply "wing it" when it comes to your approach to exercise and nutrition. You need to have a comprehensive plan when it comes to your fitness including a very specific schedule as to what days and what time of day you will exercise. You will also need to be more diligent about what you put into your body when it comes to food and drink. I can remember as a young Ranger sitting in my barracks room bored on a Saturday night just deciding at one o'clock in the morning to go on a five mile run. Not that there was anything wrong with that. In fact, it was a much more constructive Saturday night than, say, going out bar hopping would have been. However, just deciding to get in some impromptu exercise in the spur of the moment and following it up with a late-night burger run wasn't really a good approach to fitness. During those periods in my younger years when my exercise routine was not organized by others (i.e., the Army), I often neglected to even decide what specific form of exercise I was going to do on a specific day until the moment that I walked outside and began to stretch or walked into the gym. When the body is young and forgiving, you can pull this off. Not so when we age. Another factor to consider is that your time was a little bit more expendable when you were young and didn't have the responsibilities that find their way into our lives in middle age. Between my responsibilities as a husband, a father, and a physician, I have to be very diligent as to how I schedule my time. This includes how I schedule my allotted physical fitness time. A common pitfall I see is having a plan that consists of the statement, "I'm going to start getting more exercise." While that sounds great, it is basically intangible and lacks the specifics that are required to make real progress. You need to have a real plan.

Start off by planning around the number of days per week you can reasonably dedicate to your fitness. Next, determine how many hours per day you have available. Do you have a large block in the morning? At mid-day? In the evening? Or do you have multiple smaller blocks throughout the day every day? Figure out when you have free time on a consistent basis that can be dedicated to your physical fitness. Once you have allotted the time, you now have to determine what your exercise goals are and how you are going to reach them. This may involve enlisting a fitness coach. In future chapters, I will discuss the development and execution of a proper fitness plan, as well as provide specific guidance on diet and nutrition. For now, suffice it to say that neither should be attempted "on the fly"; both must be planned.

NUMBER 4: RECOVER PROPERLY

Our middle-aged bodies are not as resilient as those of our youth. Although it has always been true that fitness gains happen during the recovery phase, it is only as we age that we truly come to appreciate this. It is vital that you do everything properly when it comes to recovery. Stretching, mobility, heat or ice when needed, sleep, nutrition, supplementation, and hydration—all form the foundation for proper recovery of our soft tissues, bones and joints, and our nervous system.

If you're reading this, you have probably spent a great deal of your life focused on performance optimization. I am not asking you to abandon that now. I'm asking you to recognize that with longevity optimization as your priority, you can still have the best of both worlds. By making longevity optimization your "North Star" in guiding your journey, you can consistently reach higher levels of peak performance while avoiding both short- and long-term injury. This is the path of the warrior-athlete.

TAKEAWAYS

- Embrace the lifestyle of the warrior-athlete
- Use the wisdom of your life experience to guide you in your approach to optimization of both performance and longevity. (Use what you have learned and listen to your body.)
- Recognize the collective wisdom that is out there, and don't be afraid to try new things. (The old ways aren't always the best.)
- Do not sacrifice long-term health for short-term goals. (Life is a marathon, not a sprint.)
- Failing to plan means planning to fail. (Be specific about your exercise and nutrition, and don't allow yourself to think you can "wing it.")
- Allow yourself to recover properly. (This may take longer and require more discipline than in your youth.)

✳ CHAPTER 2 ✳

AGING

Let's take a step back for a moment and closely examine what happens to our bodies when we age. If muscles are still muscles and bones are still bones, why are our bodies different as we get older? Why do those exercise and recovery techniques that worked well for us in our youth no longer achieve the desired results? In this chapter, I'm going to go over the effects of aging on the different body systems. I will illustrate the changes that naturally occur with age and what we can do to compensate for those changes. I also hope to show you that many of the medical conditions that most people assume to be normal byproducts of aging are not normal at all and are actually quite avoidable.

I once had a patient who was approximately my age, and when I asked him if he had any chronic medical conditions, he said to me, "You know, just all the usual stuff that comes with age." When I inquired as to what he meant by that, he said, "High blood pressure, diabetes, high cholesterol—all the stuff that everybody gets when they reach 50," and he chuckled. It dawned on me at that moment what an incredible disservice the medical profession has done by allowing people to believe that these serious, potentially life-threatening, typically avoidable conditions are normal aspects of aging.

This story illustrates that there are two ways in which the medical establishment has failed. First, the medical profession as a whole has been too timid in getting people to take ownership of their own health. Physicians have become enablers, as people lead sedentary lifestyles and eat all the wrong foods. The concept of personal responsibility as it relates to one's health has become alien to most people. People blame their genetics, they blame fast-food chains, they blame their busy schedules, and they blame big government for not coming to the rescue. Not enough people in the medical community have the courage to step up and tell people to take personal responsibility for their own heath. The second problem is that the healthcare profession continues to facilitate bad behavior by offering "cures." Rather than tell someone with high blood pressure or high cholesterol to modify their diet and get some exercise, doctors prescribe pills. They give them a "cure." Instead of telling someone who is morbidly obese to stop eating fast food and start doing burpees, their doctor offers them a surgical solution to their weight problem. Quick and easy shortcuts to health are extremely alluring in our fast-paced "drive-thru" society, and the medical profession bears a large portion of the blame.

Now, I'm not saying that diet and exercise are the panacea 100 percent of the time. On the contrary, many people eat healthy foods and exercise regularly and still require medications or even invasive procedures through no fault of their own. But this is *not* the majority of cases. Aging and its effects are very real, but they are not an excuse to be lazy! Although the passage of time is inevitable, the effects of aging are highly variable.

With that, let's get back to the task at hand and discuss how aging affects our bodies' systems and exactly what that means as it applies to both our performance and longevity.

THE CARDIOVASCULAR SYSTEM

The human body contains 60,000 miles of blood vessels. This network accommodates a constant flow of "traffic" 24 hours a day for our entire lifespan. As we age, our blood vessels lose elasticity and become less pliable in a process known as *atherosclerosis*, commonly referred to as "hardening of the arteries." Poor diet (especially high cholesterol) can compound this problem by causing the buildup of "plaques" that further narrow the vessels and make it even more difficult to push the blood through. What results is increased strain on the heart as well as elevated blood pressure. Another byproduct of the loss of elasticity is that the vessels have decreased ability to "squeeze" when they need to. Have you ever noticed that getting up from a sitting position too quickly will make you lightheaded? This is a result of the arteries in your lower body not constricting efficiently in order to keep the blood in your brain as you rise. Atherosclerosis is very difficult to reverse, but it can be slowed down and even halted.

Genetics plays a role in atherosclerosis, as do the normal effects of aging, but there are three highly impactful factors that are within your control: smoking, elevated cholesterol levels (specifically the "bad" cholesterol), and high blood sugar. If you smoke, quit. Quit right now. I cannot emphasize this enough, as it is probably the absolute worst thing anyone can do to their body on a voluntary basis. Full disclosure: approximately once a month, I smoke a cigar. Cigars are *not* a safe alternative to cigarettes by any means, but there is no data suggesting that moderate/occasional use contributes to ill health effects in the manner that chronic cigarette smoking does (this isn't an excuse). As I mentioned in the previous chapter, I used to have a daily chewing tobacco habit, which is likely as bad or worse than cigarette smoking as far as health impact. I am thankful every day that I was able to quit, which was extremely difficult. There is no such thing as safe and healthy tobacco use, just as there is no such thing as safe and healthy consumption of sugary soda, which is why moderation is key. When something becomes a daily habit or, even worse, a dependency, that's when you start to inflict serious damage to your health. The role that diet plays, especially as it applies to cholesterol and blood sugar levels, cannot be overstated.

Now, in addition to elevated blood pressure, increased work on the heart, and decreased capability to rapidly adjust to postural changes, there is also a decrease in blood flow to areas with narrow capillary beds. This is the primary driving factor in erectile dysfunction in men. Decreased blood flow to muscles means less oxygen and nutrients being delivered during activity. In severe cases, this can manifest as "claudication," or muscle pain secondary to lack of blood flow and oxygen. Even in moderate cases, the decrease in blood flow will mean that greater emphasis must be placed on warming up and stretching (in that order) than was necessary earlier in life when blood flow was still at optimal levels.

Something else that you must consider: as your blood vessels become stiffer, plaque deposits increase, and blood pressure rises, you create weak spots in those vessels that could rupture and bleed during periods of elevated pressure. This can result in a hemorrhagic (bleeding) stroke or a ruptured aneurysm. Additionally, plaques can become dislodged and block arteries, causing a heart attack or ischemic (no blood flow) stroke. Whenever you hear the disclaimer, "Always consult your doctor before starting exercise!" this is why. These can kill you or leave you severely disabled. I cannot emphasize this enough. SEE YOUR DOCTOR BEFORE EXERCISING! And cease exercise if you have any of the symptoms associated with heart attack or stroke.

If you are cleared to conduct aerobic exercise, it, combined with good nutrition and smoking cessation, is one of the best things you can do for your cardiovascular health. Start slow, be consistent, and know when to stop, but get some exercise if your doctor says it is safe to do so. This is the tonic of youth when it comes to cardiovascular health.

THE DIGESTIVE SYSTEM

As I stated, there's an entire chapter ahead on diet and nutrition, so that won't be covered here. The point of this section is solely to illustrate some of the changes to the digestive system that occur with age.

In my youth, I could eat a bowl of three-alarm chili and wash it down with a cappuccino then lay down for a nap without feeling even a second of discomfort. Now, I carry Tums in my pocket all the time. As we age, we become more prone to gastroesophageal reflux disease (GERD), which can ultimately lead to more serious problems that include ulcers and even cancer. It isn't so much that our digestive tract becomes less tolerant of certain foods, but more so that food moves through the system more slowly. This manifests in various ways.

You may have noticed as you have gotten older that your appetite for breakfast isn't as voracious as it once was. We grew up in a time in which breakfast was emphasized as "the most important meal of the day" and now it seems (at least, to me) like work to choke down what once would have been considered standard fare. Not only does the aging digestive tract move more slowly, but it also takes a little longer to get going in the morning. It's like the car you need to let idle on a winter morning. A way to help with this is to drink 8–16 ounces of water as soon as you wake up. This has *numerous* health benefits, and you will see me reiterate it multiple times throughout this book. The benefit I want to address now is that it gets your digestive tract moving with something easy before you try to follow up with a meal. Like driving your car on an easy downhill slope before really giving it the gas, getting your digestive system moving also means helping out with that first morning bowel movement. There are tons of jokes out there about how middle-aged and elderly folks are very preoccupied with their bowels, but we all know those jokes are only funny because they're based in fact! Constipation is a *major* issue as we age. You don't even want to know how many times I have had to manually disimpact an octogenarian who had not had a

BM in days. That isn't a pleasant experience for the doctor or the patient, so you want to avoid it. Drink water! (You're going to get tired of me saying this, but I'm going to keep saying it.)

Bottom line: you need to be more selective about what you put into your body as you age. Your stomach and your intestines—not to mention your liver—have been through a lot. While you once could kick ass on Pop-tarts and chili dogs, you just can't do that anymore.

Another important fact: your body stores fuel as fat and as a substance called *glycogen* (the main storage form of glucose in our body). As we age, our storage and utilization of glycogen is less efficient. This means the days of going all day without eating and still having energy to do an evening workout are probably gone.

Final note on your digestive system: get your screenings for colon cancer, and get a colonoscopy if/when your doctor recommends it. This is a very common but very treatable form of cancer that you should take seriously at age 40 and above!

HORMONES (THE ENDOCRINE SYSTEM)

Age-related hormone and hormone-receptor changes could be a whole book in itself, and it has been. Long story short, your metabolism slows down as you age. What that means is that your body will have more of a challenge converting food to energy and will store more fat. This is caused by a combination of your body becoming less efficient at producing hormones and the hormone receptors on the target cells becoming resistant to their effects. Hormones are responsible for a myriad of functions. Some are *anabolic* (function in building, repair, and "fuel" storage), while others are *catabolic* (function in the breakdown and transfer of "fuel" from storage to use). Ideally, there is a delicate balance. When we are young and growing, or entering young adulthood, anabolic hormones prevail. As we age, catabolic hormones tend to have more pronounced activity.

Our pituitary gland secretes *Human Growth Hormone (HGH)*, which functions exactly how the name implies. It is a driver of anabolic metabolism in building muscle and repairing tissues. HGH levels peak during puberty and then decline, first sharply to around age 30, then slowly but steadily over the course of a lifetime. HGH receptors throughout the body also develop some resistance as we age. Good sleep is *vital* to maintaining optimum levels of HGH function, as it releases in "pulses" as we are sleeping, building and healing our muscles and tissues as we recover from the day before. This is why adequate sleep is a must and becomes even more important as we age.

The *thyroid gland*, which plays a major role in total body

metabolism, is more likely to function improperly with each passing year of life. If levels are too low, you may feel sluggish and cold and gain weight. If levels are too high, you may feel hot and jittery and have weight loss that you cannot explain. Having adequate levels of iodine in your diet is important for thyroid function, especially as we age. Make sure to have your thyroid levels checked during your annual bloodwork—more frequently if thyroid disorders run in your family.

The pancreas produces *insulin*, which is your body's primary anabolic hormone, responsible for transporting glucose (sugars) *into* the cells where they can be either stored for later in the form of glycogen or used as fuel immediately. Even when the pancreas continues to function normally, aging cells throughout the body can develop "insulin resistance," which makes the glucose transport into the cells less efficient and keeps blood sugar levels higher (contributing to atherosclerosis and a multitude of other problems). This means that diet becomes more important as we age!

Cortisol, released by the adrenal glands, elevates as we get older. Known as the "stress hormone," it affects weight, mood, libido, and an array of bodily functions. Chronically elevated cortisol can make you feel "puffy" and sluggish and manifests as weight gain in the form of increased body fat. Conversely, another adrenal hormone, *aldosterone*, decreases with age and hinders our ability to conserve water. Getting proper sleep, avoiding stress, limiting alcohol consumption, and consuming adequate water are all helpful when it comes to changes in cortisol and aldosterone levels.

On the cellular level, tiny *mitochondria*, which are often referred to as the "powerhouse of the cell," decrease in both number and function. This affects all other cellular functions, whether we are talking about skeletal muscle or neurons (nerve cells). Your cells are just not generating the same level of energy that they were in your youth. Also affected with aging is an enzyme called *adenosine monophosphate-activated protein kinase (AMPK)*. AMPK plays a key role in cellular health, function, and longevity. It is especially prevalent and important in muscle cells. Some studies have shown a link between AMPK and exercise adaptation, as well as age-related decline in function. Resveratrol, found in fruits, nuts, and dark chocolate, has been shown to boost AMPK function.

For some, the best answer to these hormonal changes may be prescription medications in the form of supplemental thyroid hormone, medications to control blood glucose, or others. However, lifestyle, diet, exercise, sleep habits, and even some natural supplements can be adequate to impact hormone levels and their functions. Healthy habits also boost cellular metabolism and longevity.

SKIN (THE INTEGUMENTARY SYSTEM)

Everyone needs to take care of their skin, especially as they get older. Skin is our largest bodily organ. It is our first line of defense against disease, regulates temperature, and provides sensory input about the environment around us.

As we age, our journey through life leaves its tracks across the roadmap of our skin. Battle scars, sun damage, laugh lines, and crow's feet all tell the tale of the path traveled on the way to our seasoned years. The changes of age on our skin are the focus of an entire multi-million-dollar industry, and the centerpiece of the medical practices of many healthcare professionals. With age, our skin becomes thinner and less elastic, as does the layer of fat and connective tissue beneath it. Skin maintains less moisture, becomes more fragile, and heals more slowly than it did in our youth. Sweat glands decrease in function, which affects our ability to regulate temperature during exertion.

If you are fair-skinned like me (a ginger), you likely have a lifetime of accumulated sun damage. Even if you aren't among my pale brethren, you should still be concerned about skin cancer. You *must* get a proper skin cancer screening at least once a year. It is easy and painless and will ensure that you detect any problem spots early when they are more amenable to treatment.

Make skin care a daily routine. It isn't about vanity (although that's part of it); it's about health. Practice good hygiene, apply sunscreen and moisturizer, and eat a healthy diet rich in antioxidants and supplementation of trace minerals, such as zinc (vital for skin and collagen health and healing). If you learn to think of your skin as a vital organ and treat it as such, you will be much better off health wise.

THE GENITOURINARY SYSTEM

Even more common than jokes about middle age and bowel movements are jokes about middle-aged bladders. In discussing hormones, I mentioned the decrease in aldosterone production as we age, and this causes of increased urination. Loss of bladder elasticity also contributes to more frequent urination, as does the enlargement of our prostate gland.

Our kidneys lose some of their functional units (called *glomeruli*), and atherosclerosis decreases blood flow to the renal tissues. The ultimate effect is that more work is being performed by fewer glomeruli and with less efficiency. In diabetics and those who have more severe atherosclerosis, this functional decrease can be drastic and eventually result in total kidney failure—another great reason to keep your blood sugar under control and drink plenty of water.

It is no secret that the male prostate gland begins to enlarge in our 40s. This makes it more difficult to completely empty your bladder as it increases the pressure that is required to expel urine. Also, our risk of prostate cancer goes up with every year of life and approaches 80 percent by age 80. It is extremely important that you get an annual urinalysis to check kidney function and blood tests to monitor your *prostate-specific antigen (PSA)*. Also, be sure to talk to your physician about regular prostate exams.

Do not let the increased frequency of urination allow you to avoid fluid intake. This is not an excuse to get behind on the hydration curve. However, you may need to decrease your consumption of liquids during the hour or two leading up to bedtime to decrease the number of times you need to wake to relieve yourself. This is all the more reason to have that bottle of water at the bedside to drink the moment you wake in the morning. If the increase in frequency becomes too problematic or causes you to start to have accidents, you need to seek medical help. You may require medication or, in some cases, a procedure called a *transurethral resection of the prostate (TURP)* to alleviate symptoms. Your growing prostate, less efficient kidneys, and less-stretchy bladder are also good reasons to avoid too much caffeine and lay off the sugary drinks/foods.

Testosterone is a natural anabolic steroid. Ninety-five percent of our testosterone is produced by the Leydig cells of our testicles. As we age, testosterone production declines. This can manifest as decreased muscle mass, tiredness, increased body fat, exercise intolerance, and diminished libido. Because the chemical signal that tells the testicles to produce testosterone originates in the pituitary gland, which is adjacent to the hypothalamus in our brain, studies have shown there is a possible relationship between testosterone deficiency and both traumatic brain injury (TBI) and shifting sleep schedules. This is especially relevant to those of us with military experience, as TBI is common, and we tend to spend long periods of time on "reverse cycle" (sleeping during the day and conducting missions at night).

Natural methods to maintain testosterone levels include clean eating, exercise (with strength training), and proper sleep. There is conflicting data on whether or not natural supplements or specific foods can boost testosterone. For me personally, in my early 40s, I noticed a decrease in energy and libido, and some weight gain in the form of fat that I couldn't seem to take care of. A check of my testosterone revealed that my levels were lower than they should have been, and I began weekly injections to supplement my testosterone back to normal levels. Even with healthy lifestyle, diet, and exercise, I still require *exogenous* (not made by my own body) testosterone. Low testosterone, how to manage it, and whether or not you need it is the subject of many books for both the professional and the layperson. If you have concerns about your testosterone, my advice to you is threefold: maintain a healthy lifestyle, consult your doctor, and read *The Testosterone Replacement Field Manual* by my good friend and colleague Dr. Andrew Winge.

THE MUSCULOSKELETAL SYSTEM

Sarcopenia is a fancy medical term for the loss of muscle mass that occurs as we age. The aforementioned prevalence of catabolic hormones over anabolic hormones majorly contributes to this. Muscle glycogen stores are decreased, meaning less "on demand" energy is available when the muscles need it. The number of mitochondria in each individual muscle cell decreases with age, so there are fewer "engines" pushing the load. The lower level of testosterone I discussed previously also contributes to the loss of muscle mass. This is cyclical, as less mass and less use of those muscles then tells your body to make less testosterone. This is all the more reason to continue with resistance/weight strength training as we get older. Bundles of muscles are surrounded by fibrous fascia and connect to our bones with tendons. Both fascia and tendons become less elastic as we age and heal more slowly. This is why it is vitally important to get some blood flowing and stretch before exercising.

The bones and joints of our axial skeleton are under pressure each and every day as we move about. Our skeletal system maintains our posture, protects vital organs, acts as the leverage point for muscular contraction, and is the site where new blood cells are formed. Decline in bone and joint health is common as we age. You can probably remember as a kid that it seemed every person over age 50 had "arthritis," "lumbago," or a "bad knee." For me personally, a lifetime of walking in combat gear has wreaked havoc on the cartilage in my knees and herniated discs in my spine.

Even when we are younger, cartilage in our joints and the ligaments that hold our bones together are slow to heal. As we age, this becomes even slower, and the tissues are more brittle, which places us at greater risk for a sidelining injury. This means we need to train smart, not be reckless, and know when to slow down.

As our bones are stressed during exercise, microscopic fractures occur. In a healthy person with adequate Calcium, vitamin D3, and vitamin K2, new bone matrixes will form that will then be even stronger. This strengthening of bone was described by the 19th century surgeon Julius Wolff, and the function has come to be described as "Wolff's Law." *Wolff's* Law theorizes that bones will adapt to added stress and demand placed upon them and remodel/rebuild accordingly, assuming the person is both healthy and also has the nutritional components and the time to heal.

If the breakdown of bone is too rapid for the system to keep up, or if the person lacks the elements to rebuild bone, then the aforementioned microfractures are never adequately repaired, and bone breaks down. Even in the healthiest person, there is a degree of bone degeneration over time due to normal physical stress and metabolic/hormonal changes. This is partly why we get shorter as we age and is also the cause of the skeletal changes we physicians see on the x-rays of elderly patients. The good news: good diet and exercise can help. The bad news: once damage occurs, you are probably about ten years behind. This is another good argument for proper diet, supplementation, and strength training *consistently* over the course of your life.

THE NERVOUS SYSTEM

Our nervous system is essentially who we are as people. Our intelligence, personality, and ability to process information and react to it, as well as all of our autonomic functions that we take for granted, are all manifestations of our nervous system. With aging, nerve cells atrophy, and waste products accumulate as those cells become less efficient at "cleaning up." Nerve impulses can travel more slowly. We lose brain mass as we age and can also develop plaques and lesions associated with cognitive decline and dementia. For diabetics or anyone with blood glucose in a chronically elevated state, peripheral nerve damage can result, causing pain and altered sensation in the hands and especially in the feet.

The keys to brain and nerve health as we age are all the things I have repeatedly discussed in the arena of healthy living. Furthermore, I am a firm believer in the "use it or lose it" philosophy: if you aren't being mentally stimulated and continuing to learn, then you are facilitating neurological decline. Continue to learn new things, always. By this, I am not only referring to book learning but also to learning new skills and practicing new physical tasks to keep all the areas of your brain and all your peripheral nerves in a state of continuous development and growth. Learn a second language, take up yoga or a martial art (make it Brazilian Jiu Jitsu!), write a novel, or learn to juggle. The moment you stop challenging your nervous system to adapt and improve, it will think you're done, and it will get lazy. Don't let your brain get lazy!

THE IMMUNE SYSTEM AND HEALING

As we age, our ability to fight off infection declines, and our *immune system* takes longer to recognize a threat and respond accordingly. Many of the immunities we developed in childhood, either through vaccination or contracting illness, no longer function optimally. For this reason, we often find that we must be re-immunized against diseases such as pneumonia and shingles. Our immune system is also responsible for detecting and eliminating abnormal cells. As this ability becomes impaired, our risk of cancer increases. Injuries hurt more (at least, it seems that way) and heal much more slowly—not only because of the adverse effects on the mechanism of healing but also the overall decrease in blood flow. Boost your immune system in the same ways you stay healthy (diet, exercise, get fresh air and sunshine, consume vitamin C and D3 and zinc), and get regular checkups to stay up to date on all immunizations, including the flu shot.

The genetic component of our longevity is dictated by something called *telomeres*. Telomeres are like caps on the ends of our DNA strands. Every time our DNA replicates itself and a cell divides, the telomeres get a little shorter. Think of telomeres like the roll of tickets you would get at the carnival. As you go on each ride and try your luck at each game on the boardwalk, you tear off a ticket. When you're out of tickets, your carnival trip is over. We have a fixed quantity of telomeres for a lifetime. They are our tickets for the big ride. Everything that has been identified as "bad" for you (smoking, obesity, stress, etc.) has been shown to decrease the length of your telomeres and, therefore, to decrease both quality of life and lifespan. Want healthy telomeres? Then live healthily. Studies have shown that we can slow down the rate at which the ticket stubs get pulled off by making healthy choices. As of the writing of this book, I have been made aware of ongoing research into peptides that have shown promise in actually *lengthening* telomeres and possibly prolonging life. There is also research into hypobaric oxygen therapy for the same purpose. I will be paying close attention to all of the research into telomere preservation and lengthening as it continues to develop.

I hope that what you take away from this chapter is not doom and gloom or that aging is just a big shit sandwich we all have to eat. On the contrary, this can be the absolute best time of your life, as long as you learn from all you have done before and heed the advice I provide you in these pages. As I stated previously: although the passage of time is inevitable, the effects of aging are highly variable. Be the outlier!

TAKEAWAYS

- Our bodies *are* different than they were in our youth. (That doesn't mean we cannot perform, only that we need to be mindful and modify our approach.)
- Chronic disease is *not* a "normal" part of aging. (Life doesn't cause diabetes and high blood pressure; *lifestyle* does!)
- Proper diet and exercise can increase both lifespan and quality of life. (You can have better quantity *and* quality if you make smart choices.)
- Don't smoke. (Smoking is probably the worst thing anyone can voluntarily do to their body.)
- Heart health = body health. (Proper exercise directly impacts heart health, which improves overall health.)
- Watch what you eat. (This is important always but even more so as we age.)
- Hormone function declines with age, but a healthy life-style can help counter those effects. (Eating healthy and

staying active help keep your hormones in the optimal range, even as we age.)

- We lose muscle and bone mass with age. Weight/resistance training is vital for musculoskeletal maintenance. (The *norm* is to lose muscle and bone mass with age, but this *can* be avoided!)
- Never stop learning, and keep your brain stimulated. ("Use it, or lose it.")
- Take precautions against illness. (Get vaccinated, practice a healthy lifestyle, etc.)
- Healing and recovery take longer than in our youth. (Patience comes with age, so take advantage of that patience and do not be in a rush.)

✳ CHAPTER 3 ✳

SLEEP

It may seem odd that I am putting a chapter on sleep at this point in the book, as opposed to covering it after other topics, so it occurs at the "end of the day," so to speak. I am doing that for a few reasons. First, I want you to think of this guide as a way to start a new chapter in your life and doing that means you would start the night before, not in the morning when you get up. Second, sleep is when we truly make progress physically and when our nervous system gets to reset both cognitively and psychologically. Third, I know you are probably like me, and if I put this chapter last, you'd put the book down after the chapter on fitness to go do some burpees and might not come back. So, we are going to cover this now. Okay?

Sleep is a particularly sticky topic with me, as I have had

difficulty sleeping since I was in my teens. My time in the military and time working variable shifts as an EM Physician only compounded this problem. Consequently, I have lived the life of a sleep-deprived insomniac for as long as I can remember. While deployed and working exclusively on a "reverse cycle," I was completely dependent on prescription sleep aids and had to wean myself off of them when I got back home. It took time and effort to return to a regular sleep schedule. Over the course of my military career, the Army subjected me to two different sleep studies and ultimately gave me various recommendations that proved to be largely unhelpful. So, like most things, I decided to study it myself and find my own answers.

I am sure it isn't news to you that we spend one-third of our life sleeping. That is a lot of time to be sure. I cannot remember how many times I have heard people talking about all the things human beings could accomplish if they did not require sleep. Well, we do require it, so there's no point in lamenting it. It is a physiological necessity. However, I propose that instead of thinking of it as lost time, think of it as *bonus* time that we get to take care of our mind and body. What if you could dedicate one-third of your time to working out or meditating? Would that sound like a pretty sweet deal? Well, you can, and you do, each and every night when you go to bed. As you sleep, your body is transforming the work you put in during the day into mental and physical gains. Tissues are repairing themselves to be stronger than they were before, and your brain is cleaning up its RAM to run more efficiently.

During your waking hours, even if you are not extremely active, multiple metabolic processes are going on at all times. It is only during sleep that your body can divert the bulk of its resources to the vital processes of protein synthesis and tissue repair. Think of how difficult it would be to change your spark plugs while your car is rolling down the street, even at an idle. Virtually impossible, right? The same is true for your body. Once you have "shut down," your body's maintenance systems can divert their attention away from the moment-to-moment functions of wakeful activity and concentrate on restoring and repairing.

(I won't bore you with describing the stages of sleep and what they mean. The definitions lack universality, and you don't need to know them.)

During the deeper phases of sleep, systemic vascular resistance drops, not only secondary to the fact that you are lying down, but also because of a decrease in what is called "sympathetic tone." This means that the heart has less work to do, while blood flow to many of your muscles and tissues actually increases. This increase in blood flow allows for the removal of any toxins or waste products from those tissues, while increasing the amount of oxygen and essential nutrients being delivered. As I touched on in the previous chapter, Human Growth Hormone (HGH) releases in pulses throughout the sleep cycle, stimulating breakdown of fat, building of protein, boosting the immune system, and multiple other functions vital for health. All these actions combine to promote bigger, stronger muscles, and a leaner, healthier body by morning.

The increased blood flow also carries fluids to the areas that need it the most. Cells that worked hard during the day and gave up a lot of their intracellular fluid must now replenish. Likewise, your joint spaces and vertebral discs "squeeze" out a lot of fluid as you move around during the day, which is then restored at night. I am sure you have heard that you are at your tallest first thing in the morning. It is true. That is because your cartilage "re-hydrates" as you sleep. You may also notice that your feet and ankles swell during the day and that the swelling has subsided by morning. The period of rest and lying flat allows your lymphatic system to move that fluid out of your lower extremities and back into circulation. What all this fluid shifting means, in a nutshell, is that your circulating blood volume is at its most concentrated in those first waking hours of the morning. If you went to bed pushing 40 weight oil, you wake up pushing 60 weight oil. Remember that 8–16 ounces of water I said you needed to drink as soon as you wake up? That's how you are going to stay ahead of the hydration curve throughout the day! Don't start out of the gate with your heart pushing extra hard to move thick, viscous blood through your vessels. Thin the mix before you engage in activity. You'll thank me.

Restful sleep isn't just for healing of soft tissues. It is equally important, if not more so, for your nervous system. Think about how you feel when you do not get adequate sleep. That is your nervous system protesting that it did not have an adequate rest period. As cognitive issues are even more common as we age, it is a vital aspect of brain health that you get the proper amount of restful sleep.

Our brain and spinal column are surrounded by a clear fluid known as *Cerebrospinal Fluid (CSF)*. Throughout the day, waste products build up in our CSF, including potentially toxic proteins known as beta-amyloids. At night, while you sleep, the CSF is "flushed out" and cleansed by what is known as the glymphatic system. The elimination of these beta-amyloid proteins is important, as their buildup has been linked to cognitive decline and conditions such as Alzheimer's dementia.

In addition to the biochemical cleansing that occurs in your brain during sleep, it is also the period in which everything you learned from the previous day gets stored in an organized fashion. All of the episodic memory you have temporarily stored in the hippocampus is transferred to permanent memory in the cerebral cortex. Your brain also "time stamps" and organizes your memories. Think of it like this: right before you go to sleep, you hand your brain a basket of dirty laundry. During the night, your brain washes, irons, and neatly hangs up your clothes, so you have ready access to them in the future and you don't have to dig through the dresser drawers to find them.

Just as I like to think of the *real* fitness gains occurring during sleep, that is also when I become better at Jiu Jitsu, shooting, and practicing medicine because everything I learned that day is organized and chiseled in stone while I sleep.

The amount of sleep that a person needs will vary depending on the individual and what they are doing, activity-wise. The general consensus is that most people need somewhere between seven and nine hours of sleep. When we are in our teens and growing, we actually require more than that (and none of us get it). Traditional teaching states that, after age 60, the amount of sleep required declines. I do not believe this to be true. I think the amount of sleep that most people over 60 actually *get* declines, and I think people have just come to accept the short end of the stick on this. The reasons for this decrease in sleep as we age is multifactorial, but decrease in melatonin production by our brain plays a key role.

Melatonin is a hormone produced by the pineal gland which regulates our sleep-wake cycle. In addition to telling us when to sleep and contributing to making us "sleepy," melatonin is also an extremely potent antioxidant that scavenges free radicals from our system as we sleep. It is often used as an over-the-counter sleep aid to treat insomnia, and I highly recommend its use as a supplement for those who may need it.

Now, in order to get that eight hours of restful sleep, you need to determine what time you need to get up and back up 11–12 hours. So, for the purpose of this explanation, let's say you have determined that you need to wake up at six o'clock in the morning, so we are kicking off our "routine" around six or seven o'clock the night before.

Most of the literature supports not eating anything substantial between two to three hours before bedtime. You certainly should avoid anything heavy/fatty/spicy within three hours of laying down to sleep, and you shouldn't have any caffeinated beverages with dinner. I would even go as far as saying no caffeine after two in the afternoon. I love coffee, but you have to limit your intake due to the *diuretic* (increased urination) effect and the over-stimulation, especially if you want to perform well while still getting that "boost" from it when you need it. Over time, you can build up a tolerance and even a dependence on caffeine, which means it won't work as well, and you will want/need more of it. Set the two-hour mark (seven o'clock in the evening) as a "hard stop" to stop eating anything. As you finish up your last meal, two to three hours before bed, I highly encourage you to take a couple over-the-counter chewable antacids. As I have stated earlier, we are more prone to reflux as we get older, particularly when we lie down in the evening. It is best to head this off in advance by neutralizing the acid at the source. Antacids have the added benefit of acting as a calcium supplement as they chemically break down in our stomach and give the body what it requires to build/repair bone during the night. In our middle-aged years, the two hours prior to bedtime is also when we should really back off on our liquid consumption, to decrease the number of trips to the bathroom required overnight.

The two-hour window is also when you should not be doing any strenuous exercise. For those of us that go to evening martial arts classes (or yoga, Pilates, etc.), this can be challenging. Strenuous exercise in close proximity to bedtime will make falling asleep more difficult. I will admit, sometimes I am driving home from Jiu Jitsu at 8:30 while drinking a protein shake, knowing that I have an early work day the following morning. But I try not to make that a habit. Whenever possible, keep to the "two-hour rule" as it applies to exercise and eating. If you are doing some type of evening workout, making it a flexibility or mobility routine is probably the best idea. Keep the high intensity stuff for earlier in the day. I am fortunate at this stage in my life to have a pretty flexible schedule, especially in the morning, but I know not everyone has that luxury.

Also, during this two-hour period you should start to "wind down." This means you are reducing your stimulation and relaxing: no action movies, no loud music, no news programs, etc. You also need to cut your "screen time" on your phone, tablet, or computer during this time. Remember melatonin? Well, the blue light emitted by electronic screens will inhibit melatonin release and may cause insomnia. If you must use your device, then you should adjust it toward the red spectrum and away from blue. Many of the newer devices have a setting to do this automatically. The hours before laying down to sleep are not the time to be on social media or looking at annoying news sites. This can and should be a time for relaxing reading and quiet reflection. Personally, I like the feel of a traditional book in my hand during the evening hours. Remember, the things you read will be fresh in your hippocampus as you nod off to sleep and primed for transfer to permanent memory, so you want that information to be constructive, not frustrating or banal.

Your preparation to go to bed should be a calming ritual and should follow a pattern. By sticking to the pattern, your body will learn that this is the "shutdown sequence" and will transition more readily into slumber. Before starting your ritual to prepare for sleep, plug in your phone and leave it on the nightstand or wherever you keep it at night. Leave it there! It shouldn't be the last thing you see or touch before going to sleep. Brush/floss your teeth, and wash your face as a minimum, even if you don't shower before bed. If you don't sleep in the buff, then wear something loose fitting, light, and comfortable. Whatever you do, do not sleep in the same sweaty underwear you have been wearing for 12 hours. It's not only uncomfortable; it's flat-out disgusting and unsanitary.

The ideal temperature for sleeping has been determined in multiple studies to be right around 65 degrees Fahrenheit. For those of us in Texas, that can present a challenge, unless you don't care about your electric bill. There are a few ways you can "augment" your sleeping environment that will help and do not entail running the air-conditioning full blast. In addition to changing your mattress every ten years (and choosing one of quality and appropriate firmness), you should cover it with a mattress topper that is changed every three years. Choose one that allows airflow and will keep you cooler. Of all the areas of your life that you might chose to pinch pennies, your bedding shouldn't be one of them. This includes quality sheets and comforters that match the season, not just your bedroom décor. Ceiling fans are nice, as long as you have one that is functional and not simply decorative. If you do set up a portable fan, I recommend not facing it directly at you. Position the fan in a corner pushing air down a wall to cycle the air in the room. This is preferable to having the fan blowing on you all night, drying out your mucous membranes. Finally, I recommend a double layer of shades and thick "black-out" curtains on the windows. Not only will they keep out light, but they will also act as a barrier to ambient noise and provide a level of temperature insulation. If your bedroom windows face the south, you may want to add a layer of reflective window film, as southern-facing rooms tend to be warmer. The result of these steps will be a cool, dark "cave" of sorts, which sounds awful but is actually a great place to sleep.

An added step that you may require is placing a white noise machine in your bedroom. Depending on where you live and what types of noises you have to deal with, this may be a necessity. In multiple studies, white noise has been shown to lower the amplitude of human brainwaves. Lower amplitude brainwaves are consistent with drowsiness and restful sleep. Separate clinical studies have shown that white noise helped hospitalized patients fall asleep faster and achieve deeper, more restful sleep.

Side note: I know some people are concerned that a white noise machine could prevent them from hearing a noise in the night that requires a response, such as an intruder or a crying child. Speaking from my own experience, by keeping the volume on my white noise machine on the lowest setting, this has never been an issue. Several times, I have been able to respond to concerning noises in the night that were in no way "masked" by my white noise machine, and I have been using one for over ten years now.

Now that your "cave" is prepared, it is important that you understand that it is designated for two purposes only: sleeping and intimacy with your partner. Your bed is not a place to eat, watch television, surf the internet, etc. You must establish this habit so that your brain and body form an association that this is a place of sleep and rest. Some light reading before turning out the light is acceptable, but don't plan on balancing your checkbook or answering emails. Sex and sleep. That's it.

Your final step before climbing into bed is to place that 8–16-ounce container of fresh water on the nightstand. I don't want you going to the fridge or the pantry to fetch it when you wake up; I want it right there in arm's reach. Remember that!

I recommend that you plan on being in bed, with everything "turned off" at 9 p.m., nine hours before you have to get up. This "extra" hour gives you ample time to fall asleep initially, as well as get back to sleep if anything in the night wakes you (a trip to the bathroom, a noise, an ache or pain that rouses you, etc.). Knowing you have this extra hour will also mean you are more relaxed and that you don't feel like the eight-hour clock is ticking down the moment your head hits the pillow.

Now, once you are in bed, you want to fall into a deep and restful sleep. This has always been a problem for me, as it is for around one-third of American adults. The pressures of career, finances, family, etc., all weigh heavily on the mind when the lights go out. You need to let that go. Think of it this way: is anything you are going to do in your bed at 9 p.m. going to "fix" anything? Is losing sleep while thinking about your problems going to serve any purpose? Of course not. As falling asleep has been a lifelong issue with me, I did a great deal of personal research and discovered a way to make it easy.

Hypnagogia is the name given to the transitional state of consciousness between wakefulness and sleep. Thomas Edison had a bit of an obsession with this phase and referred to it as the "Twilight State" in his notes. The hypnagogic state describes the brief period as you are falling asleep when you experience vivid hallucinations. You may experience brief flashes of light, random images that last for only a second before transforming to something else entirely, or the sound and sensation of the ocean around you. This is the time where you may suddenly wake with a start to catch yourself from an imagined fall that seemed very real. When I first read about the hypnagogic state and recognized the description as it related to my own experience, I began to wonder if I could somehow induce that state purposefully. With a little practice, I found that I could cycle imagery in my conscious mind, which my unconscious mind would then takeover after a few minutes. By quieting the parts of my mind that wanted to dwell on the details and difficulties of my everyday life and gently probing that part of my mind that acts as a doorway to a more relaxed state of consciousness, I was able to fall asleep quickly and easily. I know this might sound a little "out there," but trust me on this.

In bed in your "cave" with your eyes closed, breathe deeply and begin to cycle images in your mind. The images should be calming, such as trees blowing in the wind or a gently flowing river. Avoid anything with too much movement or action, such as vehicles or moving animals. Allow the image to hold in your mind only for a second; just long enough to fully manifest and recognize it, and then let it go. Transition immediately to the next image (an iceberg, a field of wheat, etc.) and continue to do this until you feel the images start to control themselves. Do not resist, but instead allow those images to cycle on their own. You may feel that they begin to become more vivid as this occurs. That is your subconscious mind taking over the steering wheel and driving you toward your destination: deep and restful sleep.

If the imagery technique doesn't seem to work for you, then simply close your eyes and watch the moving balls of light gliding across your eyelids. Focus on them and try to influence the shapes. Picture this like a controllable "lava lamp" in front of you. Once you find that you can control their movement, let yourself breathe deeply and relax, continuing to watch while allowing them to move on their own. Do not let any thoughts other than those moving lights encroach into your conscious mind. Leave behind everything that required your attention during the day, and let yourself relax.

If my technique doesn't work for you and you are still having trouble falling asleep, I encourage you to do a little research on your own and try different techniques until you find what works for you. There are multiple YouTube videos, apps, and meditation programs that you can find offering various techniques. Whatever ultimately works isn't just to help you fall asleep initially but also to fall *back* asleep if you find yourself awake in the night. It is not uncommon to awake in the wee hours and wonder about your car's "check engine" light or an upcoming work deadline. Don't do that. Whatever technique you find to help you to induce a more relaxed state of consciousness, go back to it. Focusing on any topic, positive or negative, will activate the more highly cognitive centers of the brain and induce a more wakeful state of consciousness.

Even with the techniques I described, you may still have difficulty either falling asleep or staying asleep. This is a big reason why so many people turn to prescription or over-the-counter sleep aids. As I stated previously, I have had issues with dependence on prescription sleep aids. These are not long-term medications, as they have some serious side effects over time. A far better option in terms of both physical and cognitive health is natural supplements to help relax and achieve restful sleep.

I mentioned taking antacids with your evening meal for the benefit of both reflux control and calcium supplementation. This isn't really going to help with sleep, but timing-wise, I would categorize it with your "evening supplements" all the same. Here are some other evening supplements that I have found to be beneficial when it comes to sleep.

MELATONIN

I have mentioned already melatonin and melatonin supplementation. Melatonin is probably the most common over-the-counter natural sleep aid that people take. Between 1–3 milligrams of melatonin is considered to be an optimal dose. My advice is to start with 1 mg and see how you do. I personally take 3 mg before bedtime.

MAGNESIUM

Magnesium is a very important mineral that many people are deficient in. Magnesium is vital for electrical activity in both the heart and the brain. It is also helpful in relaxing muscles and opening up the terminal airways of our lungs, thereby increasing oxygenation. Most studies indicate that between 100 mg and 350 mg is extremely helpful in maintaining sleep. I tend to recommend dosages just a little higher, as people are typically deficient, and your body will have no trouble eliminating excess as long as your kidneys are functioning normally. (If you have abnormal kidney function, you should consult your doctor before taking magnesium.) I take 400 mg before bedtime.

VALERIAN ROOT

Valerian root extract has long been used as a natural sleep aid and has been clinically proven to be effective. I have found that a dosage of 400 mg can be quite effective in promoting sleep.

L-TRYPTOPHAN

You are probably familiar with *L-tryptophan*, which is a naturally occurring amino acid. It is classified as an "essential" amino acid, as your body cannot synthesize it, and you must get it through diet or supplementation. It is found in large quantities in turkey meat and is the culprit responsible for the late afternoon Thanksgiving nap. I have found doses of 500 mg to 1,000 mg to be the ideal range and take 650 mg myself.

My advice on all sleep aids and supplements is to first consult your doctor, then start with one supplement at a low dose and move up as needed. Then, add more supplements as necessary. I also recommend you take one to two weeks off every six to eight weeks to maintain sensitivity and continue to get the optimal benefit. Finally, even though it is "over-the-counter," you should avoid sleep aids that contain *diphenhydramine* (Benadryl). Studies have shown that diphenhydramine actually prevents you from reaching the deepest and most restful stages of sleep in a timely fashion. You may fall asleep more quickly, but it will not be the quality sleep that your body requires.

As the focus of this book is men in the fifth decade of life and beyond, I would be remiss if I didn't at least briefly discuss sleep apnea. If you have difficulty sleeping that has progressed as you have aged, I highly recommend getting a referral for a sleep study, especially if you are overweight and/or have unexplained high blood pressure. There are three types of sleep apnea, so let's briefly discuss them.

Obstructive sleep apnea (OSA) is caused by excess soft tissue in the pharynx and is often associated with snoring. Side sleeping and weight loss can be helpful, although a CPAP machine is the ultimate treatment in most cases. *Central sleep apnea (CSA)*, which I have, is a disorder where your brain occasionally "forgets" to breathe while you sleep. CPAP is also helpful for central sleep apnea, as is avoidance of alcohol, opiates, and other substances that can profoundly depress brain function. *Complex sleep apnea* is a poorly defined complex set of symptoms that is considered to be a combination of OSA and CSA. It is somewhat controversial as a diagnosis and requires a more nuanced approach when it comes to treatment. The bottom line: see a physician who is board-certified as a sleep specialist if you have any questions or concerns or if the simple techniques I have outlined do not prove helpful in achieving restful sleep.

If you can't get adequate sleep, all of the clean eating and physical exercise in the world is not going to be helpful. If you happen to be one of those people who can get by on minimal sleep and still feel physically strong and mentally sharp, then count yourself lucky. For the rest of us, we may need a little extra help to recharge overnight and awake refreshed and ready to meet the day.

When you do wake up in the morning, do not stand up right away. Take a moment to stretch and breathe deeply, and let your body adjust. Move to a sitting position with your feet on the ground, but don't stand up just yet. Reach for that 8-16 ounces of water on the nightstand, and drink it all before you rise to your feet. Replenish the fluids that your body needs, wake up your digestive tract, and allow your vascular system to equilibrate as you drink. Then, get up, and not only meet the day, attack it!

TAKEAWAYS

- Sleep is vital to brain and body health. (Working out and eating right mean nothing if you don't get good sleep.)
- No caffeine after 2 p.m. (Getting through the afternoon without it will be difficult the first couple of days, but you'll be better off.)

- Plan your sleep schedule backwards from the next morning to the evening prior. (Decide when you need to be up and go back 11–12 hours.)
- Start "winding down" two hours before bed. (Stop eating food, restrict fluids, and decrease stimulation and screen time.)
- Build your "sleep cave" (dark, cool, quiet, and comfortable).
- Keep 8–16 ounces of water on the nightstand. (You will drink it all as soon as you get up in the morning.)
- Once in bed, put your mind in a state to transition into sleep. (Displace "anchored" thoughts, and use techniques to achieve a state of hypnagogia.)
- Avoid prescription sleep aids and Benadryl. (Prescription sleep aids can cause dependency, and Benadryl can prevent restful sleep.)
- Use natural sleep aids as needed:
    ◦ Melatonin
    ◦ Magnesium
    ◦ Valerian root
    ◦ L-tryptophan
- Talk to your doctor about a sleep study. (Sleep apnea is common beginning in the fifth decade of life and beyond.)

✳ CHAPTER 4 ✳

DIET AND NUTRITION

Note: for the purpose of simplicity, I use the common term "calories" in place of the term "kilocalories" (Kcal).

This is a difficult topic for me to tackle. Basically, I like food. I like junk food, desserts, and everything that you are told is bad for you. I like soda, and pizza, and cheeseburgers, and all that crap. Getting my diet in line has always been the most difficult part of fitness and health for me. I love to exercise, so that's easy. What is *extremely* challenging is not celebrating every kickass workout with tacos! The truth of it is diet is probably more important than your workout routine. So, if your diet sucks, then you just aren't going to see the full benefit of working out. The old saying, "Fitness happens in the kitchen, not the gym," really is true, as much as I sometimes wish it weren't.

Before the switch could really flip for me, I had to start looking at food as fuel and to recognize that everything I put into my body would affect my performance and my overall health. If you are putting garbage fuel into your gas tank, your carburetor will clog, your spark plugs will foul, and you will stall while driving uphill. It makes no difference that you put that turbo charger on your engine if low octane sludge is what you are putting in the tank. Nothing that I am saying should be news to you, and I am sure you have heard it all before, but have you really taken it to heart?

Spoiler alert: There is no shortcut. No quick fix. No magical diet. To really make an impact on a long-term scale, you must approach nutrition from a *lifestyle* standpoint. Think back to the chapter on performance vs. longevity, and apply that same logic to your diet. Look at your nutritional choices through the lens of the long term, not from the point of view that you want to lose 15 pounds in a month. When you look at nutrition through that short-term lens, you are susceptible to the allure of the "dark side": the crash diet.

We have all fallen victim to the siren's call of the crash diet at least once in our lives—a month before beach season, two weeks before the high school reunion, a week before our annual physical when we knew our doctor had cautioned us about our weight, etc. Drastic calorie-cutting, exclusionary diets, "cleanses," and other shortcuts to rapid weight loss certainly may work temporarily, but at what expense? Aside from the fact that we were never designed to eat like that, the bigger problem usually ends up being the psychological and physiological rebound afterward that actually causes us to put on more weight in the form of fat.

Although the keys to eating a healthy diet aren't complicated, they are elusive, so it is entirely understandable that many people find it challenging. We are bombarded with marketing for the super-mega-ultra-combo-meals with special sauce and a 64-ounce soda. In our current society, food has become quick, easy, delicious, and deadly. The Centers for Disease Control (CDC) currently estimates that just under 50 percent of all American adults are obese. That means half the country! If you look around and don't think that number is correct, it is likely because you have become so accustomed to seeing fat people that you no longer process it as being out of the ordinary.

When we were kids, eating out was a "special occasion" that happened rarely. Today, Americans eat out far more frequently, and because they want their "money's worth," they tend toward the less healthy alternatives on the menu and demand larger portions for their dollar. When I was in medical school, I had the pleasure of listening to a talk by former United States Surgeon General C. Everett Koop. Dr. Koop spoke at length on his observation that restaurant portions had increased exponentially in size over the course of his lifetime and that this went hand-in-hand with our national obesity epidemic.

The increase in portion sizes isn't confined to eating out. It has penetrated our homes as well. Dinner plates are 25 percent larger now than they were a century ago. In fact, what we now think of as a dinner plate would have once been considered a serving platter to our grandparents. Portions, and waist sizes, have gradually increased over time. Add to this the fact that we simply do not prepare meals in the same manner anymore, and you have a recipe for disaster (pun intended).

Whereas previous generations made everything "from scratch" using more fresh ingredients, our fast-paced microwavable lifestyle has pushed us more toward pre-prepared ingredients that come in a can, in a box, or frozen. The combination of larger portions, and the fact that so much of what we eat is processed food (as opposed to fresh food), means that as we have gotten older, we have eaten food that is less healthy, in larger amounts. This is the opposite of what we should be doing. So, how do we eat healthy?

Since we were kids, we have been shown the various "dietary guidelines" developed by the United States Food and Drug Administration (USDA). In health class, we learned the "four food groups" and how much of each group we should eat. In 1992, they introduced the "food pyramid," and we were told that it represented a "healthy diet." What we didn't know was that the food pyramid wasn't based in science at all but was bought and paid for by lobbyists who pushed to have it "modified," so they could sell more products. Later attempts by the USDA to revamp the pyramid made it no more scientifically valid but did make it more confusing to follow. Only recently have the USDA recommendations become even close to being correct, but they are still very skewed.

Constant disinformation, 24-hour marketing, and a fast-paced society that prizes convenience all make for a terrible environment when it comes to food. It is no wonder that we find it so challenging to eat healthy. But that doesn't mean you are off the hook. When the rubber meets the road, *you* have personal responsibility for what you put into *your* body. You are neither a victim nor a passive observer in this endeavor. Since you are still reading, I will assume that you recognize this, and that you are ready to embrace it. So, let's go.

Keep in mind that no particular set of nutritional guidelines is going to suit everyone. Age, body type, genetics, activity level—all play a role. The absolute best thing a person can do is work one-on-one with a nutritionist as a guide, especially in the early stages of the lifestyle change. But I recognize this just isn't possible for most people. Barring that, it is an excellent idea at least initially, to either keep a food log or to use one of the many available phone apps that will help you track what you are eating.

I am going to provide you with some general guidelines that have a solid foundation and have worked well for me and for others. These are guidelines only, and not a "one-size-fits-all" solution, so be aware that you may require some adjustment. (Your mileage may vary.)

Most dietary plans utilize a "top-down" approach by determining how many calories you need first and then dictating how you divide those calories up. I prefer to work from the ground up. I like to approach a nutritional plan by starting with the macronutrients you require and building from there. I have found this method to be useful because of its simplicity. In case you are not familiar with macronutrients, there are three groups: carbohydrates, proteins, and fats. Some resources list water and fiber as macronutrients, but I do not feel that is appropriate and also think it confuses things.

As I am sure you already know, carbohydrates are our body's main source of fuel, and your body can either use them shortly after ingestion, or they can be stored for later. Proteins are the building blocks that make up all the tissues of our body, muscles being the most obvious. Fats are an important source of energy and are a crucial component of all cells. Fats are also vital for synthesis of hormones and help our body to utilize certain vitamins and micro-nutrients. In my approach to nutritional planning, I start with proteins and work from there. Your protein and calorie requirements will vary based on activity, age, and goals (weight loss, weight maintenance, or weight gain), but I have a baseline that I recommend as a starting point.

My general rule of thumb is that you should strive toward consuming 0.75 grams of protein daily for each pound of body weight. So, for a 175-pound man, that equates to 131 grams of protein daily. This amount is a bit higher than the Recommended Daily Allowance (RDA) dictated by the Food and Nutrition Board of the Institute of Medicine, which recommends 0.8 grams per kilogram (0.36 grams per pound). It should be noted that their recommendation is for a *sedentary* person (which most Americans are) and doesn't take into account the increasing protein needs of age to prevent muscle loss. I think that it is important to prioritize your protein intake first and go from there, without putting too much emphasis on total calorie count. By prioritizing protein, you minimize the risk of getting "filled up" on carbs or fats before reaching your protein goals. The amount of protein I recommend is going to seem like a lot to most people. My advice is to shoot for 0.75 grams per pound as a baseline and adjust upward *if* you are doing a lot of high intensity/weight training and are trying to build muscle/gain weight. A word of caution: higher protein diets have been associated with increased risk of kidney stones, so you should consider this if you have a history of them. I also recommend consulting your doctor.

Fats are the most calorically dense of the three macronutrients (a gram of protein or a gram of carbs is equal to four calories, while a gram of fat is equal to nine calories), so you need less of them in your diet as a rule. In my younger days, I tried various "low-fat" diets, and sometimes they worked well, but the fact of the matter is you *need* adequate healthy fats in your diet for all the reasons I have detailed. Fat grams should be equal to half (½) your weight in pounds. So, for that same 175-pound man, 88 grams of fat would be the ideal amount.

Carbohydrates are the macro that most people tend to get too much of and the one that most guidelines typically allow to be half or more of the total calories consumed, which I think is a mistake. Our western diet is very high in carbohydrates, specifically "bad" carbohydrates. If you get too many, then they are stored as fat. I recommend around 1.2 grams of carbohydrates per day per pound of body weight. This number can be adjusted down or up, depending on activity level and where you are in your training cycle. So, for 175 pounds of body weight, that means 210 grams of carbohydrates per day. (This will seem like a very low number of carbs to most people. Remember: it is a baseline and can be increased as needed.)

As I said, this plan is designed from the ground up and isn't focused on a set number of calories, which is probably different from what you are accustomed to seeing. I don't like plans based on calories and have always said, "Don't count calories. Make your calories count." Although there have been times when I have kept a calorie log to reach specific goals, I try not to make it a habit, and I don't think it is easy to sustain as a lifestyle.

In case you were wondering, this plan would come out to 2,157 daily calories as a baseline, with protein making up 24 percent of the total calories (525 calories). Again, this is solely for your information, in case you care. Fat would comprise 37 percent (792 calories), and carbohydrates, 39 percent (840 calories). A quick caveat: if you are either obese or underweight, then you may consider adjusting all these amounts based off of where you want to be headed, weight-wise, as opposed to where you are currently.

Most of the guidelines out there call for baseline daily caloric intake between 2,000 and 3,000 calories based on activity level and weight goals. My plan fits right into that number but includes a lower percentage of carbohydrates than is typically recommended and slightly higher ratios of protein and fat. Again, I don't want you to concentrate on the calories; concentrate on the grams of protein as a priority, and the rest will typically sort itself out. I try to simply focus on my grams of protein and make healthy choices in the fat and carbohydrate categories when meeting my caloric needs (as determined by what my body tells me in the form of hunger and energy, as opposed to numbers). The way I determine those needs is pretty simple: if I am hungry, I probably need to eat. My credo when it comes to food is: "Never be hungry, and never be full." If I feel hungry, I eat something, but I never gorge myself to the point of feeling "full." You need to determine the difference between satiety and fullness. Satiety is when you feel you have eaten enough to normalize your blood sugar, whereas fullness is when you feel you need to loosen the top button of your pants and take a nap. Since fats and carbs tend to be the culprits when we go off the rails, keeping your protein grams in the crosshairs will make you less likely to overindulge in the other two macros. As long as you are tracking the protein, there's some flexibility in the other two depending on what you're doing. A day with a tough morning workout and an afternoon or evening martial arts class typically means larger portions of healthy carbs and fats at lunch, while a day that is more sedentary might mean less. You can adjust up or down, as long as those adjustments are based in healthy food choices.

One last note on calories: as a general rule, if you burn more calories than you eat, you will lose weight, and if you consume more calories than you burn, you will gain weight. If your goal is to gain weight in the form of muscle, or to lose weight in the form of fat, then being mindful of how much you consume vs. how much you burn off becomes more important. As I said, there have been times when I kept the total number of calories in mind, either because I was looking to bulk up in the form of lean muscle or looking to slim down by burning fat. Again, think of the amounts I give as a *baseline* for someone who is seeking to maintain a healthy weight, and you can adjust from there based on your specific goals.

Now, let's talk about your choices in how to get those nutrients. (This is far more important than the numbers.)

Red meat has gotten a bad rap, and it is partially deserved. Red meat does tend to contain more saturated and trans fats (also known as "bad" fats) than chicken or fish, but it is also protein dense and rich in iron and vitamin B12. Grass-fed beef and meats like venison or bison are healthier than the typical grain-fed (fattier) beef you are accustomed to seeing in the butcher section at your local grocery store. Data is conflicting and ever-changing on how much red meat is considered "healthy," so I am not even going to attempt to tell you how much you can or can't eat. I will say that you should attempt to get the bulk of your daily protein from fish and poultry and make that really good steak a special treat. The more you rely on fish and poultry for your protein needs, the better off you will be in terms of your cholesterol and in terms of getting healthy vs. unhealthy fats (fish contains the "good" fats). Beans, nuts, and dairy products, as well as eggs, are also good protein sources. I tend to use a whey protein supplement on most days, especially after a workout, simply because eating enough protein-rich food to meet my 0.75-grams-per-pound goal can be tiring. What you should *avoid* is processed meats. Pretty much every study shows that eating processed meats, such as salami and bacon, is unhealthy. Sadly, this means eating less bacon. (I love bacon.)

Remember, you need to get that 0.75 grams of protein per pound of body weight, so that means reaching for protein-rich options when you snack. Another big advantage of high protein snacks is that the sensation of satiety (not feeling hungry) lasts longer than with typical healthy carbohydrate snacks such as fruit. I am a huge fan of almonds and almond butter, as well as cheese cubes and yogurt. Sardines are an amazingly healthy high-protein snack, as well as a great source of vitamin D, calcium, and Omega-3 fatty acids (good for you!). Sardines are also very low in toxins such as mercury when compared to most other forms of fish such as tuna. However, the "social" aspect of eating sardines tends to drive people away (both literally and figuratively). If you like them and people around you can tolerate the smell, then I highly recommend sardines as a snack.

Speaking of healthy fats, let's talk about where to get your ½ gram per pound of body weight.

As I mentioned, fish is a great source of healthy fat. What constitutes a healthy vs. unhealthy fat could fill an entire book in and of itself, and I really don't think we need to get that far into the weeds. For the most part, unsaturated fats tend to be healthier than saturated fats, but this isn't always the case. As a rule, fats from animal protein (other than fish) tend to be the "bad" kind, whereas fats from plant sources are of the healthier variety. Avocados are a great source of healthy fats, and one avocado contains about 20 grams of good fat. Many nuts are great sources of healthy fats, with pistachios being one of my favorites. Cooking with healthy oils such as canola oil or extra virgin olive oil will provide you with some good fat as well. Another great option is to add some coconut oil to your coffee. Coconut oil is a rich source of medium-chain triglycerides (MCTs), which show promising results in providing a spectrum of positive health effects. Not only does coconut oil provide healthy fat, but it tastes great, staves off hunger, and has been theorized to form fat "capsules" that allow for a slow and sustained release of caffeine over time as opposed to a "jolt and crash."

There are a few different companies out there that offer snacks that provide a high quantity of healthy fats, as they have become pretty popular among those on "ketogenic" diets. Avoid butter, fatty red meat, bacon (I know; it makes me sad too), and too much dairy. If your cholesterol and triglycerides have been an issue for you in the past, you need to be working closely with your doctor to develop a plan to combat this, and your diet should reflect that plan. Keep in mind that the amount of fat I recommend is higher than most sources, including the RDA. This is contingent on you eating *healthy* fats and is not a license to eat bacon and cheesesteaks every day.

Carbohydrates are where most people get into trouble. You need carbs for energy, and they are the only thing that will replenish the glycogen in your muscles and your liver. Glycogen is a vital source of "emergency fuel" when your muscles need it. If you have ever engaged in a sudden burst of energy, such as a sprint, then you've burned glycogen to do it. The carb intake I personally target is 1.2 grams per pound of body weight, but it tends to fluctuate based on my activity. More important than the grams or calories is that the majority of the carbohydrates you consume come from sources with a *low-glycemic index*. Consumption of low-glycemic index carbohydrates will keep your insulin levels from spiking (this can cause weight gain and not the good kind), increase insulin sensitivity, and can help elevate HDL cholesterol while lowering LDL cholesterol. Green vegetables, whole grains, legumes, and certain fruits, such as apples and pears, are all considered to be low-glycemic index foods. Avoid bread, pasta, potatoes, and fruit juices as much as possible. Foods like sweet potatoes, oatmeal, and brown rice are considered to be in the "medium"-glycemic index category and are fine in moderation. Honestly, if you only take one thing away from this entire chapter, it would be that word: "moderation." The problem that we have as Americans is we have forgotten what that word means.

The key to getting these macros in the proper amounts is to eat as much fresh food as possible. If it comes in a can or box, or if you got it in the freezer section, then it is processed and probably bad for you. Lean healthy meats, healthy plant-sourced fats, green leafy vegetables, whole grains, and fresh fruits are your tickets to healthy eating. Notice, you didn't see burgers, fries, pizza, or doughnuts in there. When you do stray off the healthy path, exercise some control, and don't let it become a regular occurrence. There's nothing wrong with a well-earned bacon cheeseburger and a side of truffle fries occasionally, but it shouldn't be a daily, or even weekly, event. *Moderation*—there's that word again.

Sodas and sugary drinks tend to be a big problem for a lot of people, myself included. Don't try and fool yourself with diet sodas either, as the artificial sweeteners impact insulin secretion, as well as sensitivity, and have been linked to Type 2 diabetes. Water is what your body needs and what you need to be drinking. But if you need some flavor or carbonation with a meal, I get that (I do too). Sparkling water is a great option for a meal beverage and is just as healthy as still water as long as there is no added sweetener or sugar. Now, let's talk about how much water you should be drinking.

You have already heard me harping on getting that initial 8–16 ounces as soon as you wake up, and I am ringing that bell yet again because it is so important. Remember: you never want to wait until you are thirsty to drink. If you are thirsty, then you are "behind the curve" as we say, and believe me when I tell you that you do not want to be there. Generally, depending on your activity level, you need between ½ ounce and 1 ounce of water per pound of body weight. So, for our 175-pound man, that would mean at least 88 ounces of water consumed for a day spent in air conditioning watching television and a minimum of 175 ounces on a day spent either working outside in warm weather or a day with some vigorous exercise. Since trying to track your water consumption might prove tedious, it is best to just be drinking to the point that your mouth is never dry and your urine is a light yellow or "straw" color. If your tongue is dry or your urine is dark, then you are getting behind the curve. The short- and long-term health benefits of getting enough water cannot be overstated.

Now, a word of caution: it is entirely possible to get *too much* water and doing so can cause electrolyte imbalances that result in confusion and even seizures. If you are sweating profusely and replace lost fluid with water alone, without eating, then you are at increased risk. Sodium and potassium are vital electrolytes that we lose through perspiration and must be replaced along with water to maintain proper cellular and neurological function. Drinking water is not enough; you must also replace lost electrolytes.

Years ago, when I first started working as a Mixed Martial Arts (MMA) fight physician, I discovered that many fighters were drinking distilled water (water with the minerals/electrolytes removed) during the last week of their weight cut. Based on some bizarre form of "bro science," they were under the mistaken belief that distilled water would somehow "wash out" additional weight. The dangerous part of this practice is that distilled water will actually leech existing electrolytes out of your system. This is particularly concerning considering that most of them were restricting their food intake to cut weight and were, therefore, not replacing their lost electrolytes. Bottom line here: do not drink distilled water to stay hydrated. Contrary to some of the crazy internet claims you may see, there is no proven health benefit to drinking distilled water, and it has the potential to be dangerous. The same is true for "alkaline water"; don't waste your money. Nature made water just perfect the way it is. Trust me on this.

"Sports drinks" have become very popular, but the fact of the matter is that most are very high in sugar and don't do an adequate job of replacing lost water and minerals/electrolytes, although their advertising may say otherwise. My opinion on sports drinks is that they are fine in moderation, as long as you choose those with the lowest possible sugar content.

One thing that I have yet to mention is fiber. Fiber is extremely important, especially as we age. You need to consume between 25 and 35 grams of fiber daily to maintain good bowel health and help keep your cholesterol in check. Ideally, this should be consumed in the form of high fiber foods, such as green leafy vegetables or bran. You may find it helpful to use a soluble fiber supplement to ensure you are getting enough.

Now, the elephant in the room that we need to discuss is the *exclusionary diet*. An exclusionary diet is any diet that puts certain food groups off limits. The problem that I see with these diets is that they run contrary to science and millions of years of human evolution. Don't get me wrong: I think there are foods that we tend to eat way too much of and that most people could cut back on. And if we are talking about processed food, that is absolutely something that could be eliminated for most people. However, diets that eliminate the same food groups that human beings have consumed and thrived upon for thousands of generations are both intrinsically unhealthy and difficult to maintain. Veganism has become increasingly popular, as has the "carnivore diet" at the opposite end of the dietary spectrum.

Veganism, in my opinion, is less of a diet and more of a philosophy. At the core of veganism is the belief that animals are not a commodity put on the earth for human use. If someone comes at veganism from the point of view of that core belief, then I have no problem with that nor an argument against it. However, those who point to the vegan diet as the ideal human diet are incorrect. We are omnivores, plain and simple, and our bodies are designed to draw their nutritional needs from both plant and animal sources. Vegans require much more diligent supplementation of vitamins and trace minerals when compared to a balanced omnivorous diet. Getting enough protein on a vegan diet is also challenging, as plant-sourced protein takes longer for the body to use and must be consumed in relatively high volumes. Most of the data out there on "plant-based diets" does *not* validate veganism in as much as it shows the shortcomings of the typical western diet. If by "plant-based" someone is referring to a diet in which the majority of calories per day are derived from vegetable sources, then absolutely that is healthy. But to imply that a species which has eaten meat for millions of years can somehow become herbivorous and still thrive is misguided in my professional opinion.

A *carnivore diet*, by contrast, is a diet that is restricted to animal products and does not include vegetables. This diet has become popular with those who have food allergies to various plant products and some people with conditions associated with chronic inflammation. The problem with the carnivore diet is it can lead to vitamin deficiency, elevated cholesterol, gastrointestinal problems secondary to low fiber, poor athletic performance due to lack of available carbohydrates, and may increase the risk of some cancers. Eliminating fresh fruits and vegetables also means you aren't getting the potent antioxidants that they provide. *Antioxidants* help protect you from heart disease and many forms of cancer, among other conditions associated with what we refer to medically as free radicals. As I said before, we are omnivores, and there is no need to cut healthy vegetables and fruits out of one's diet, barring specific food allergies.

Another quasi-exclusionary diet is the *ketogenic diet*. The ketogenic diet is based on extreme limitation of carbohydrate intake to the point that your body preferentially burns fats for fuel and produces ketones as a byproduct of that fat metabolism. The scientific community is split on the pros and cons of the ketogenic diet. It has been shown to be highly beneficial in patients with refractory seizure disorders and some Type 2 diabetics that have been unable to lose weight and get their blood sugar under control using other means. In my personal experience, I have tried a ketogenic diet and was indeed able to lose fat while putting on muscle. However, I didn't feel that it was sustainable as a lifestyle, at least not for me personally. I also felt that the carbohydrate restriction had an adverse effect on my endurance. I do think that most Americans get way too many carbs (as you can clearly see by my recommendations for daily nutrition) and that consumption of processed sugars should be severely limited, but I don't advocate a ketogenic diet as a lifestyle for the long term.

The last exclusionary diet I am going to touch on is the *paleo diet*. The premise of the paleo diet is that it mirrors the dietary habits of our ancestors by avoiding processed foods and foods that "hunter-gatherers" would not have had access to in their daily lives. This means cutting out breads/grains and dairy products. Of all the exclusionary diets out there, this one is probably the most in line with what we are genetically designed to be eating as it primarily excludes foods that are products of industrial farming. However, in eliminating legumes (beans, lentils, peanuts, etc.) and milk/cheese, the paleo diet takes away some great sources of both protein and vitamins. The paleo diet isn't for me, but it may be right for you.

Most exclusionary diets tout some type of weight-loss statistic. Typically, the reason for the weight loss has more to do with elimination of processed foods and the fact that you end up consuming fewer calories by default. It is my belief, and the belief of many experts, that eating whole foods in the proper proportions is the healthiest way to approach nutrition. Eat wholesome, unprocessed foods in appropriate moderation, and you are eating a healthy and sustainable diet.

Now that I have told you how much to eat and in what forms to eat it, let's talk about how you are going to eat it. As I stated earlier, "Never be hungry, and never be full." This is important, as it will keep your blood sugar steady without spiking and without crashing, which then leads to over-eating. I recommend that you eat five to six small meals a day. I know that you have been told your entire life that breakfast is the most important meal of the day, and it should be substantial, but I disagree that it should be considered the "most important" or that it should contain the highest number of calories. I don't think it is a good idea to assault your empty digestive system with a big meal. Likewise, I don't think a massive dinner is a good idea, as you are ingesting a lot of calories right before shutting down for eight to ten hours. I eat my biggest meal of the day between noon and 2 p.m. after my workout and consider it to be my "most important" meal of the day. This provides me with protein and calories when my body needs them the most and helps me avoid the desire for a high-calorie afternoon snack. If you want to break it up as three main meals and two or three smaller snacks, that is up to you, but you should be eating something every two to four hours until you reach the two-hour mark before bedtime.

That's it. That's everything. That's "the secret." Avoid processed food, prioritize protein, eat carbohydrates with a low-glycemic index and healthy fats in moderation, and drink plenty of water. Drink if you are thirsty, and consume calories if you are hungry, but don't over-indulge. It isn't radical—it isn't revolutionary, but it works, and it is both healthy *and* sustainable.

TAKEAWAYS

- Food is fuel. (Remember that you eat to live as opposed to living to eat.)
- There are no shortcuts. (Rapid weight change is unhealthy and not sustainable.)
- Concentrate on your macronutrients. (View nutrition from the ground up as opposed to the top down.)
- Prioritize 0.75 grams of protein per pound of body weight (fish, poultry, grass-fed red meat, and vegetable sources).
- Consume your baseline fat grams equal to ½ gram per pound of body weight (fish, avocados, nuts, and healthy oils containing *unsaturated* fats).
- Eat your baseline carbohydrates equal to 1.2 grams per pound of body weight (low-glycemic index foods, such as whole grains, legumes, and healthy fruits and vegetables).
- Watch your carbs closely. (Avoid too much, and avoid higher-glycemic index foods, such as pasta, bread, fruit juices, etc.)
- Avoid processed food. (If it comes in a can, a box, or the freezer section, then it isn't for you.)

- Never be hungry, and never be full. (Eat five to six times a day but never to the point of feeling "stuffed.")
- Drink plenty of water (½ ounce to 1 ounce per pound of body weight each day based on activity).
- Avoid exclusionary diets. (They are difficult to sustain and typically unhealthy.)

✳ CHAPTER 5 ✳

FITNESS

Physical fitness and our approach to it becomes more and more important as we age. The forgiving and pliable body we knew in our youth could get away with neglecting exercise, but the aging and less flexible body cannot. Not only is exercise more important, but doing so *properly* is also vital. As I have stated, you need to have a plan, and that plan needs to be based in proven science, not antiquated tradition.

A caveat that I need to get out of the way early on: consult your doctor before beginning any exercise program to ensure that you are healthy enough to exercise without risk of death or disability!

The biggest mistakes that I see aging athletes make is that

they either try to stick to "what always worked before" or they only do what is easy for them because they think they cannot "go hard" any longer. The problem with doing what worked in our youth is twofold: first, what you were doing 30 years ago wasn't the smartest way to approach fitness (I promise); second, your body is different now, for all of the reasons that I outlined in the chapter on aging. The problem with only doing what is easy should be obvious: you aren't going to improve if you aren't challenged, not just on a personal level but also on a cellular level.

Aging athletes who are still dedicated and consistent tend to fall into two categories for the most part (with some exceptions). They are either strength athletes or endurance athletes.

The *strength athletes* are still in the gym hitting the weights, usually with their knees wrapped and their old-school lifting belts on. They tend to be broad shouldered and barrel chested with a bit of a gut. By sticking to the old-school lifting routines we learned in high school, they have reached a level of "dad strength" that others envy. The problem that these guys face is they typically have very poor endurance and are actually putting a strain on their heart with all the extra body weight they are packing. You see, your heart is like the engine of a truck in that it works harder depending on the load and doesn't care what that load happens to be, whether it is muscle or fat.

In contrast, the *endurance athletes* are those guys who are getting in a run or a bike ride every day, including an extra-long-distance event on the weekends. Unlike their strength-athlete counterparts, they maintain a low body-fat percentage and have the same waist size they had in their 30s. Endurance athletes typically lack the muscular strength required for the application of "functional fitness," meaning tasks requiring moderate to heavy lifting will be more difficult. They also may be accelerating the sarcopenia that comes along with age and indirectly shortening their lifespan. A 2016 study by Penn State showed that people over age 65 who regularly lifted weights significantly improved their longevity when compared to their peers who did not.

The common denominator in both of these groups is that they pick what they like and stick to it, without consideration for the importance of a well-rounded fitness routine. For an athlete focused on a specific competitive discipline such as power-lifting or cross-country running, that may be okay. But for a warrior-athlete focused on both performance in everyday life as well as longevity, you have to achieve balance and seek to be well-rounded. Not only is it important to work both strength and endurance but also to work on flexibility, mobility, power (different than strength), and durability. I call these *The Six Pillars of Fitness*, although none of them truly stand alone, as they overlap quite a bit.

STRENGTH

The concept of *strength* is something we are all familiar with, and its meaning is fairly straightforward. The simplest gauge of how *strong* you are is the one-rep maximum or the "max" that we were first exposed to in gym class. Although some people look at the "max" as a goal in and of itself, I see it more as a gauge that helps me determine my workout weight for that particular exercise. Although I do squats, bench press, dead lift, and many other conventional weight-training exercises, I honestly don't put a lot of thought into what my current "max" is for any of them. Early on in a new fitness program, I may determine my one-rep maximum to calculate 70 percent of that weight as a starting point for sets of 8–12 repetitions. Strength should also be viewed in two ways: *absolute* strength, which is how much weight you are lifting, and *relative* strength, which is how much you are able to lift as a percentage of your body weight. I always put more emphasis on relative strength, since I am competing with myself and not others who are larger or smaller than I am. The secret to improving strength isn't really a secret: lift heavier weights. By gradually increasing your workout weight, you build strength. Because I am lifting to improve my functional strength and not to simply increase my "max" or make my muscles huge, I never do sets of less than 8 or more than 12, and I typically do 3–4 sets of a given exercise. I find this to be a balanced approach that fits best with my fitness goals. Now, traditional *strength* training is usually higher weights for lower reps, which is what works best for *maximum strength*. Because I am more focused on repetitive strength, which overlaps with *muscular endurance* (discussed in the next paragraph), I keep to higher reps, while still using the generic term "strength" to describe these workouts.

ENDURANCE

Endurance, like strength, should also be divided into two categories: *cardiovascular* endurance and *muscular* endurance. Cardiovascular endurance is the ability of your heart and lungs to deliver oxygen to your body during prolonged physical activity, such as a long run or bike ride. Muscular endurance is the ability of individual muscles to contract repeatedly in a specific period of time, such as performing as many pushups as possible in a two-minute period. Both aspects of endurance are important to overall fitness. While a pure cardiovascular exercise such as an eight mile run will not significantly improve muscular endurance, performing muscular endurance exercises in the form of circuit training or High Intensity Interval Training (HIIT) will improve both cardiovascular *and* muscular endurance as long as you are maintaining the proper cardiovascular threshold for a sustained period of time. My aforementioned method of 8–12 reps for 3–4 sets ensures that weight training is not only addressing strength (both maximum and repetitive, with emphasis on repetitive) but also muscular endurance.

FLEXIBILITY

Flexibility is exactly what it sounds like. Unfortunately, flexibility tends to be one of the first things we start to lose with age, and it becomes more difficult to maintain and improve as our connective tissues become less pliable and do not heal as efficiently. Flexibility is typically determined by passively stretching a joint and is primarily (but not solely) a determination of the elasticity of ligaments (the connective tissue bands that hold bones together) and tendons (connecting muscle to bone). Traditionally, we have sought to improve flexibility through static stretching: forceful stretching of joints held at maximum extension for sustained intervals. In our youth, we were taught that *dynamic* stretching (bouncing) was a bad idea and could cause injury. We now know that a certain degree of dynamic stretching, when not performed too forcefully, is actually highly beneficial.

MOBILITY

By contrast, *mobility* is a function of *active* movement. Mobility is determined by a combination of muscular strength, joint health, and the elasticity of the fascia (the tissue that surrounds and covers our muscles), as well as tendons and ligaments. In other words, when Bruce Lee bent over and touched his forehead to his knees, he was demonstrating flexibility; when he kicked his leg up to strike a target over his head, he was demonstrating mobility. Performing mobility movements should always be a part of your warmup routine and can even be a workout in itself, especially if you are returning to working out after a period of rest. Yoga is amazing for working on mobility.

POWER

Power is often confused with strength, which it is not, although they certainly are closely related. While strength is a measure of how much resistance a muscle can move, *power* is determined by how quickly that resistance can be overcome. I have often used the term *explosiveness* interchangeably with power. An offensive lineman may determine his strength by how much he can squat, while his power will be better measured by pushing a weighted sled for a distance of ten yards as quickly as possible. Power is best developed by performing explosive/rapid movements. Take care when conducting any resistance exercise explosively, especially compound and/or complex movements that involve multiple muscles and joints. These types of exercises are extremely useful but can result in injury if you sacrifice form for speed. "Wall ball" throws, ball slams, jumping lunges, and over-the-shoulder sandbag throws are some of my favorite power exercises.

DURABILITY

The sixth pillar is *durability*. Durability is interconnected with all of the other pillars and balance. Whereas strength and power are largely dependent on the big muscles, or what we refer to as the *prime movers*, durability is more a function of the accessory and stabilization muscles. Most of us have neglected the durability aspect of fitness for a good portion of our lives and have paid the price with injuries. Dumbbell and kettlebell movements conducted smoothly with a single arm or with weight on one foot are great for strengthening the stabilization muscles that protect your joints, especially if you emphasize a slow and deliberate "negative" movement (typically, the downward portion of the repetition). Working single limb/side movements and performing slow and deliberate repetitions is not only beneficial, but it is also safe to perform without a spotter and means you can use less weight to get more benefit. Core exercises are also important to increase durability as they help maintain proper posture and protect you from injuring your back. Most forms of dumbbell presses, lunges, and dips, as well as "good mornings" and Turkish getups, are all excellent durability exercises.

Now, before planning your workout routine, the most important question you should ask yourself is what you are working out *for*. What are your goals? What physical tasks do you hope to accomplish? What metrics outside of the gym determine if you have reached an optimal level of fitness? If it is a number on a scale, wearing certain clothes, or looking a certain way, those aren't really good metrics.

Not that a weight-loss goal might not be important, but it is not a stand-alone gauge of physical fitness.

During my military career, the Army Physical Fitness Test (APFT) was used as an objective measurement of physical conditioning. Although it is a highly flawed test, especially as it applies to combat readiness, it is a fairly decent yardstick to assess initial fitness and determine progress. This three-event test consists of two minutes of pushups for maximum reps, two minutes of sit-ups for maximum reps, and a two-mile run for time. In Ranger Regiment, we added a fourth event: dead-hang pull-ups for maximum repetitions. If you're looking for a simple way to gauge your baseline and periodically evaluate your improvement, this might be an easy way for you to do so. As I said, not the best test out there, but it can be conducted alone, with minimal equipment, and can be completed in less than an hour.

Personally, my own fitness routine is geared toward improving my performance in Brazilian Jiu Jitsu (BJJ) and Mixed Martial Arts (MMA). I gauge where I am on the spectrum of fitness by my ability to effectively spar at full speed for multiple rounds in a 30-minute period with no more than a 1-minute break between rounds. Striking, takedowns, and fighting for position all work muscular and cardiovascular endurance and provide feedback on my strength and power. My ability to perform complex moves against a fully resisting opponent is a direct reflection of my mobility and power, and how I feel the next day tells me a lot about my flexibility and durability. By training in combat sports, I am getting a real-time functional assessment of my fitness. If you were to watch my typical fitness workout, it would look a lot like what you have come to expect from a "CrossFit" workout, but it isn't. Don't get me wrong: I am not against CrossFit. I actually think the CrossFit movement has done a lot to promote fitness and that high-level CrossFit practitioners are exceptional athletes, but I don't think it is right for me for a couple of reasons.

Those who attend a CrossFit gym will go to the "box" and perform the "Workout of the Day" (WOD) posted for everyone to see. This may be a WOD that the gym management decided on its own, or it might be the one dictated by the franchise. Either way, all clients are generally expected to do that day's WOD or a variation. The plus side of this is that you can work out and compete as a group. The downside is that it may be comprised of exercises that do not target your specific fitness goals or that do not take your abilities and fitness level into account. The other thing that personally keeps me from doing CrossFit is that the WODs often involve complex movements performed to muscle failure, which in my experience can be a recipe for injury. I prefer to have a plan that is more customized and takes my personal fitness journey into account, one where my coach knows my limitations and concerns. Thousands of people have achieved great results with CrossFit, so if it works for you, then by all means, stick with it. It just doesn't happen to be for me.

Bottom line: figure out where you are and where you want to be when it comes to fitness. This isn't a journey you are going to be able to take without a map and a reference for where you are starting out. Speaking of road maps: there is also a huge advantage to having a guide in the form of a fitness coach. Whereas there is only so much that I can go into in this chapter and only so much you can learn from the resources that are out there, a coach is trained in this arena and can help you navigate a comprehensive fitness plan that will help you meet your individual goals. In my early 50s, I made the decision to enlist the help of a fitness coach, and it was one of the best decisions I have ever made. Working out is a skillset, just like anything else. Would you try to learn martial arts or competitive shooting solely from a book or a video? Of course not. While open-source resources are great adjuncts, they aren't a substitute for expertise and proper training. I highly recommend you enlist the help of a fitness coach, even if only during the first few months, to establish a solid foundation.

Another aspect of assessing your fitness starting point and charting your progress is determining your *resting heart rate* (RHR) and *maximum heart rate* (MHR). To determine your RHR, sit comfortably for at least ten minutes, preferably early in the day, then feel the pulse in your wrist with your fingertips and count for one minute. Stimulants such as caffeine and nicotine can affect your resting heart rate, as can various medications. Over time, as your fitness improves, you will see your resting heart rate decrease as your cardiovascular system increases in efficiency. The "standard" method to determine your MHR is to subtract your age from 220. This technically means that for every year you age you would drop one beat per minute of maximum heart rate. Obviously, this isn't 100 percent accurate. I prefer to use the method determined by the HUNT Fitness Study, which is *211 - (0.64 × age)*, as I have found it to be more precise.

When we are young, our MHR is relatively high, while our RHR tends to be low (less circulatory resistance and a young, healthy heart). The difference between our RHR and our MHR is our *heart rate reserve* (HRR). The HRR is how much "room to play" we have. At age 30, with a low RHR (say, 60 beats per minute) and a high MHR (approximately 191), the HRR is around 131. As we age, our HRR narrows. Using me as an example, my resting heart rate is 51 beats per minute, and my maximum heart rate is 176 (211 - (0.64 × 54) = 176). By subtracting my resting heart rate from my maximum heart rate, I can determine my HRR is 125. As you can see, we don't have as much reserve as we age, at least not on paper. You can also see, because I work out enough to keep my resting heart rate low, that gives me more room in my HRR compared to my age-group peers, and I am not all that far behind a 30-year-old.

Once you have determined those three numbers, it's time to figure out your three "zones." Some sources go as far as breaking down heart rate into five zones or more; I don't think you need to go that far. We aren't really concerned about the zones on the "low end" when you are at rest or doing something light. I focus primarily on three zones: fat burning, aerobic fitness, and anaerobic training. You should also be aware that there is some disagreement about the exact cutoffs of the zones. In truth, the numbers have some variability, and it isn't like some internal switch "flips" at a certain heart rate. Keep in mind, these zones are mostly important when you are doing sustained activity that is geared towards endurance. I don't have a zone that I target when doing strength training, although I do wear my heart monitor whenever I exercise, no matter what type of activity that happens to be.

FAT-BURNING ZONE

Your fat-burning zone is between 50 percent and 75 percent effort. This is computed using your HRR and adding your RHR. Example (for me): $0.5 \times 125 + 51 = 114$, and $0.75 \times 125 + 51 = 145$. That means that maintaining an exercise heart rate between 114 and 145 (50 percent – 75 percent) keeps me primarily burning fat as fuel in a process known as *beta oxidation*. This is a zone where you can sustain the effort for extended periods of an hour or more. Keep in mind, although you are primarily burning fat for fuel, the actual calories expended is lower in this zone than in the aerobic or anaerobic zones. This is where you want your heart rate to be on that really long run/jog or bike ride and where you will build endurance as it relates to sustained activity. However, you shouldn't expect tremendous improvement here, especially if that is the only zone you target during workouts. If exercise is new to you, then this is a good place to hang out for a while, until you are ready to challenge yourself.

AEROBIC-FITNESS ZONE

Your aerobic fitness zone is between 75 percent and 85 percent effort. Example (for me): $0.75 \times 125 + 51 = 145$, and $0.85 \times 125 + 51 = 157$. Therefore, my aerobic fitness zone is 145 to 157. This is the zone where you start to really "feel it." When performing endurance training, this is the zone that I strive to spend the most time in during exercise, especially for workouts under an hour. Keep in mind, the closer you are to the 75 percent mark on the lower end, the more "fat burning" you are probably doing. As your heart rate increases, your metabolism shifts away from fat as a fuel and moves toward carbohydrate consumption in the form of *glycolysis*. At the same time, the amount of calories per minute that you burn increases as your sustained heart rate gets higher. Depending on where you are in your fitness journey, you should spend between 20 and 60 minutes in this zone to increase cardiovascular endurance.

ANAEROBIC TRAINING

The anaerobic training zone is everything above 90 percent effort. Using the same method, $0.9 \times 125 + 51 = 164$. This is the "hardcore" training zone where you really push yourself but where you don't need to spend a lot of time. It is in the anaerobic zone that you feel the edge of your fitness envelope. This is the zone where you burn energy exclusively from circulating blood glucose and stored glycogen. This is also the zone where your body produces lactic acid as a byproduct of that glucose metabolism occurring without adequate oxygen (that's why is it is called *an*aerobic). I consider between four to six minutes in this zone per workout (collectively, not necessarily continuously) to be indicative of a solid workout.

You may have noticed that there is a gap in there of five percent effort between the aerobic fitness zone and the anaerobic training zone. I like to think of this mini-zone between 85 and 90 percent as a "sweet spot." This aerobic-anaerobic threshold zone is a "mixed bag" where my body is getting energy primarily from glycolysis as it transitions away from beta oxidation. This is an area where I feel that I make a lot of performance gains, but I don't spend as much time there as I do in the aerobic zone, as it just isn't sustainable. Over time, you will find that you can spend more and more time comfortably in this zone as your fitness improves.

The "Gold Standard" for determining your thresholds/

zones and getting the most accurate assessment of your fitness is through a *VO2 Max test*. VO2 Max stands for the maximum rate of oxygen consumption measured during incremental exercise. Professional athletes and Tier 1 Military Operators use this test to gauge their level of fitness and track their progress. Many high-end gyms and health clubs have this test available for their clients, but I don't think you necessarily need it unless you just have a burning desire to know what your VO2 Max is.

Knowing where your zones are and tracking how much time you spend in them is important if you are taking your fitness seriously. I highly recommend a good heart monitor be worn during every training event. Another good idea is a "smart scale" that not only accurately tells you your weight but also utilizes electrical impedance to determine your body-fat ratio. This will help you determine if you are working out properly by burning off body fat and increasing or maintaining muscle mass. This will make the numbers on the scale mean a little bit more than just pounds.

Okay, so now that you know the six pillars of fitness, the reason you are working out, and your zones, the next step is figuring out how many days a week and how many minutes per day that you have available to work out. I recommend that you try and avoid more than two days off in a row, as that is when you start to lose some of the progress you have worked so hard for. So, if you decide that you can only commit to three out of seven days per week, it would be better to work out every other day as opposed to three days in a row with a four day break. Also, if you determine that the work week is just too busy, you may have to work out Saturday and Sunday, and then do what you can to get in brief, 30-minute workouts a couple of days during the week, possibly in the evening or during a lunch break. Personally, my shortest workout is between 30 and 45 minutes, and I make it a point to try and never go over an hour and a half. I just don't think you need to go longer than that for a "gym workout." If you are doing some cross-country stuff or an activity that is longer, that's fine, but I just don't think you should typically be spending more than 90 minutes in the gym working out. (If you spend your entire life in the gym, it kind of defeats the purpose of being in shape to live a longer and better life.)

A quick side note: there has always been a lot of debate on whether or not you should work out at home or go to an actual gym. The argument in favor of working out at home revolves around time constraints and convenience, while the argument against has to do with distractions and limitations on equipment. I will say that I have a lot of home workout gear and I do both, although 80 percent of my workouts take place in a gym away from home. I like having access to a wider variety of equipment, and I also feel like going to a gym forces me to hold myself accountable. Something about paying for the membership and traveling all the way there flips the switch in my head and makes me say, "Okay, I came all the way here, so I need to make it count!" Ultimately, it has to do with your individual personality, your finances, and what you do or do not need for your specific fitness plan.

In my opinion, four to five days per week of serious exercise (with a combination of active and passive recovery days) is ideal, although I do know some people who train all seven and have no issues with over-training (freaks of nature). I think it is better to plan to work out as many days as possible, and then when life gets in the way and you end up with an unscheduled rest day, you aren't missing out too much. For this reason, my schedule is typically five hard workout days, one active recovery day, and one passive recovery day. My coach and I structure my workouts so that I am doing a very similar routine for three to four weeks and then changing it up. This keeps me from getting bored and sloppy and forces me to challenge myself. I know there is a lot of debate around the validity of "muscle confusion" or "shocking," and it isn't something I really care to dive into. I will say that simply from the perspective of staying motivated and keeping workouts from being boring, it is a good idea to switch things up. In my 30s, I would go for months and years doing "chest and arms day," "back and biceps day," and "leg day," or some other similar variation. Not only did it not provide a well-rounded workout, but it was boring! I like working out to be fun and to keep me mentally engaged. I detest the idea of mentally "checking out" while I am exercising since I think one of the benefits of fitness is to be able to maintain mental sharpness while under physical strain. Allow me to illustrate my current workout structure as an example, that you can either use, modify, or ignore.

First off, I should point out that I start almost every gym workout with five minutes on the assault bike, jogging, or jumping rope, followed by stretching. By warming up first, you get the circulation going and "grease" your joints prior to stretching. Do not stretch while cold! Also, on any day that I am doing resistance movements (i.e., weight training) I do *supersets*, which means I alternate back and forth from one exercise to another. In other words, I might do 10–12 repetitions of goblet squats, rest 30 seconds (no more), do 10–12 cable flys, rest 30 seconds, and back to goblet squats for a total of 3–4 sets of each. Supersets allow you to move quickly from one exercise to another and maximize your time and effort in the gym. There are many ways supersets can be structured depending on what muscles/groups you are working out and what your goals are.

I should also point out that two to four days a week I am doing some type of martial arts training in the evening, so those days have two workouts and are more challenging. Just ahead, I will talk about which days those are, what I do, and how it relates to my "gym workout" on those days.

Monday, regardless of the previous week or the weekend, I concentrate on mobility and durability. Typically, this means my usual warmup and stretch, followed by actively moving through motions that will challenge my muscles in their range of movement: dive bombers, plank walks, wall walks, kick throughs, Russian twists, knee tucks, flys, get-ups, and lunges among others. I do these exercises first as they provide additional warmup and prepare me to work durability. As I said earlier, durability involves a lot of single-side/single-limb movements, such as dumbbell presses, weighted lunges, "Supermans," core exercises, and BOSU ball exercises. Any movement that seems to challenge your ability to maintain balance is probably a good durability exercise. Nothing I do on a Monday is extremely dynamic or explosive but instead is slow and deliberate. There is also a strength component to many of these movements.

Tuesday is strength day. I love Tuesdays because I get to do "old school" weight lifting like squats, dead lifts, military presses, etc. After warming up and stretching, I do paired supersets of the basic push-pull exercises we are all familiar with. As I said, I typically perform 3–4 sets of 8–12 reps and increase the weight by around 5–10 pounds each week, for however many weeks I am performing that exercise (typically 3–4). I do my best to really push to muscle failure on this day or get as close to it as safety will permit. This provides improvement in maximum strength, repetitive strength, and also muscle endurance. Tuesday night, I go to Brazilian Jiu Jitsu (BJJ) for two hours, doing warmups and drills, learning new moves, then sparring for 5-minute rounds during the final 30 minutes of class.

Wednesday is typically an active rest day for me. This can mean yoga, a mountain bike ride, stationary bike, a light jog, or some light sparring. My goal on this day is to keep moving, while not straining, strength-wise, nor getting my heart rate any higher than the lower end of my aerobic zone. Unlike other days of the week, I try not to do two workouts on Wednesdays. (I have a short chapter on recovery up ahead.)

Thursday is power day. I am really getting three for one on Thursday since working power also means working repetitive strength and endurance. Once I am warmed up and stretched, I like to do "clusters" of three to five different power movements either for a specified number of rounds or for as many repetitions as possible (AMRAP) in a given time period: push-ups, burpees, pull-ups, kettlebell swings, box jumps, sand bag throws (personal favorite!), ball slams, etc. These are explosive but controlled movements, alternating exercises. Depending on how it is structured on that day, I usually perform two separate "clusters," followed by a cool down. Thursday evening is another BJJ class.

Friday is a real ass-kicker. Friday is all about muscular and cardiovascular endurance. My goal on Friday is to keep my heart rate in the higher end of my aerobic fitness zone and work in and out of the anaerobic zone. This doesn't just mean running or biking, as I prefer to structure it more as an "around the world" where I am moving from exercise to exercise, much like the "clusters" the day prior. In addition to the assault bike, ski machine, and rower, I also like to work weighted movements that appear slow but keep the heart rate up like front rack carries, sled pushes, etc. This workout often takes the form of what you probably know as High Intensity Interval Training (HIIT). Friday's workout is usually a long one, around an hour and a half of "work." Friday evening, I usually train two hours of Thai boxing or MMA, so I am pretty worn out by the time my head hits the pillow on Friday.

Saturday is a rest day (for obvious reasons), but I still stay active since this is usually a day to do something outdoors with my family. Keeping moving, even on rest days, is important. Also, what is the point of all that working out if your off day is spent on the couch?

Sunday is another form of a HIIT workout, but I also use it as both a "carburetor cleaner" to get me going after my Saturday off and as a diagnostic tool to see where I am, fitness-wise. I will do one of two things on Sunday, depending on my mood and what else I have going on. At home, I will do Thai boxing with sprawls on my heavy bag, either ten each of two minute rounds or seven each of three minute rounds (depending on how good I feel). This is a hardcore HIIT workout, where I use a "coaching" MP4 file played on a speaker to tell me what to do and keep me moving. (If you are interested, it is the Bas Rutten MMA "All around fighting" file.) My heart rate will increase progressively over each round and return almost back to baseline between rounds during a 1-minute rest period. This is a high-yield workout for spending time in the aerobic-anaerobic threshold and the anaerobic zone. If I have more time available, I will head to a local MMA gym for an hour of "open mat" sparring, grappling for six minute rounds with one minute rest between. Both of these workouts are a great endurance, mobility, and power routine that give me an idea of where I am on the fitness spectrum.

In the chapter on recovery, I will talk more about what exactly that entails as well as go into the concept of "de-loading" and how often that should occur. I don't think it is necessary for you to mimic what I do for my routine, only that you understand the principles of a well-rounded fitness program and how you should approach it. That's one of the many reasons I am not getting too terribly specific. My workout may seem too strenuous or too light for your taste, depending on where you are on the fitness spectrum. Again, consult with a coach, or look for a resource that outlines a workout program geared toward your individual goals, using your current state of overall health as a starting point.

One thing that I cannot stress enough is that you must be consistent in your approach to fitness. I talked previously about this and how working out in "bursts" is a recipe for shortcuts and injuries. Think of it as a mathematical formula: Consistency/Time = Results or $C/T = R$. It is far better to work out 20 minutes a day for 4 days a week over the course of 20 years than to work out for 90 minutes, 6 days a week for a few months at a time. Be consistent and make it part of your lifestyle, and you will see results over time. This is true of literally *anything* in life.

A parting thought to finish up this chapter: don't skip leg day! In fact, I actually believe that every day is leg day. Leg strength, power, endurance, flexibility, mobility, and durability are literally and figuratively the foundation of total-body fitness. Neglecting your legs will lead to problems throughout your kinetic chain. Legs are the key to punching power. Legs feed the wolf. Don't skip leg day.

TAKEAWAYS

- Consult your doctor before starting an exercise program. (These aren't just words; they really are important.)
- Determine exactly what your fitness goals are. (Being "in shape" is too vague to be helpful.)
- Consider an athletic trainer or coach. (Expert advice will make your fitness journey easier.)
- Formulate a well-rounded fitness program (considering

strength, endurance, flexibility, mobility, power, and durability).

- Determine your Resting Heart Rate, Maximum Heart Rate, and three zones. (This is key in knowing if you are exercising effectively.)
- Use specific performance and body metrics to gauge your improvement. (You cannot manage what you aren't measuring.)
- Consistency/Time = Results.
- Don't skip leg day.

✳ CHAPTER 6 ✳

MARTIAL ARTS

In my opinion, the practice of martial arts is one of the most beneficial things a person can do to ensure overall wellness. A *real* martial art is grounded in the principles of effective self-defense, physical fitness, self-reliance, honor, and respect. (Notice, I said a *real* martial art, as there are several fake ones out there.) All of these contribute to legitimate self-confidence (very different from *ego*), while at the same time translating well into every other aspect of your life.

One of the many benefits of training in martial arts is that it simultaneously provides a fitness workout and fitness assessment. All six pillars of fitness are put to the test in a practical fashion. The practice of martial arts relieves stress in a way I don't think any other activity can match, while adding a valuable tool in life's toolbox in the form of providing a means of self-protection.

With notable exceptions, many serious martial artists are long-lived and maintain health and vitality well past middle age. Unfortunately, many also have chronic musculoskeletal injuries from over-training or training improperly in their youth. For this reason, I think it can actually be a *good* thing to start martial arts later in life (although, truth be told, I wish I had begun practicing seriously at a much younger age. Yeah, I am contradicting myself, but nobody is perfect). With the patience of age comes a more balanced approach, and without the invulnerability of youth, we are forced to embrace proper technique over brute force and raw athleticism.

Just like with fitness, you need to ask yourself what you want out of martial arts. Personally, I cannot comprehend why someone *wouldn't* want to be able to defend themselves and their loved ones in the event of a physical altercation, but some people study martial arts for different reasons, and that is fine. If you prefer to look at martial arts as a form of physical activity and meditation or a celebration of a proud lineage of those who refined the art over the course of generations, that's okay. To each his own. What is dangerous is those who practice martial arts with the *intent* of practical self-defense yet practice in a way that completely fails to provide that capability. These people walk around each day with a dangerous level of false confidence in their ability to deal with violence, similar to those who carry a firearm every day and think that just having a gun is some type of magic talisman that will keep them safe. Don't get me wrong: I have carried a gun virtually every day of my adult life, and I am a huge advocate that responsible adults should carry. But there is a saying: "If you carry a gun, but can't fight, then you're just someone else's holster."

Those who practice martial arts consisting of "forms" or "katas" (choreographed patterns of martial arts movements made to be practiced without a partner) and forego actual sparring and pressure testing in realistic situations are fooling themselves about the practicality of what they are doing as it applies to self-defense. If that type of thing translated to fighting ability, then every housewife who did "Tae Bo" back in the 1990s would have gone on to become UFC champions. To really be proficient in the realm of self-defense, you must pressure test everything you learn through realistic sparring. It is only through sparring that you peel back the weaknesses in your techniques and definitively expose the effectiveness of what you are doing at its very core. Again, if you are looking to practice martial arts as a sort of alternative to yoga, then by all means, do so. But if you want a true assessment of your ability to defend yourself in a physical altercation, then you need to be getting on the mats, or in the ring, or in the cage and going full speed to see if what you have learned actually works or if it is what we like to call "Bullshido."

On the opposite end of the spectrum, from the "overly gentle" martial arts, are those that make claims about their practitioners being instruments of extreme lethality. I have a hard time taking any martial art seriously if it makes claims such as, "Our techniques are too dangerous for MMA. They are made for fighting in life or death situations." Typically, that is the reason given to explain why you don't see any of their practitioners represented among the ranks of successful MMA fighters. These are usually "systems" that rely on "finishing moves," such as eye gouges, groin strikes, biting, etc. The problem with these is exactly as I illustrated previously: they are incapable of being pressure tested. It is impossible to *really* practice these crippling or lethal moves, and therefore, you will never truly know if they are effective or if you are doing them properly. The fact of the matter is the reasons these types of schools don't produce UFC fighters is because what they teach is simply not effective.

Also, I am personally not a fan of any place that teaches ancient weapons or "stick fighting." Do you carry nunchucks or fighting sticks in your pocket? Then why learn them? I am pretty sure a bo staff is too long for the trunk of a car, and I seriously doubt you can get a pair of sai through airport security on vacation. Tradition is great, and if you want to study something like that as a link to history, then do so. But don't think for a moment that your ability to dance with a sword with a red ribbon tied to the handle translates into the ability to defend yourself in the real world.

So, where does that leave us? What martial art should you practice? Full disclosure, I am a practitioner of Brazilian Jiu Jitsu (BJJ), and I consider it to be the best choice for multiple reasons. But there are many others out there that can also be considered worthwhile. Muay Thai is highly effective, although I have to say that sparring at full speed, even with headgear on, can be dicey as we age. I participated in a Muay Thai "Smoker" (an in-house double elimination tournament among the students) in my mid-40s, and I won. It took me a few days to recover, and my official government passport photo has a black eye as a result, but it was worth it. Although I still train Muay Thai and MMA, I put more time and effort into BJJ and don't do as much full-speed sparring in the striking arts as I do in grappling. I feel that BJJ is the most well-rounded and most useful martial art when it comes to self-defense (*traditional* BJJ, not *sport* BJJ). Oftentimes, the effectiveness of a particular style depends more on the instructor/academy than the martial art itself. Finding the right school and avoiding a "McDojo" can be tricky, but I have some tips.

Do some online research. See what people are saying about

the place. If you notice all the reviews are written within a couple of days of one another, those are friends of the owner and are not reliable. Research the instructors, and make sure they don't have criminal records. (You would be shocked to know how many convicted criminals are teaching martial arts. Unfortunately, this includes sex offenders.) Websites for the school should not only tell you the belt rank of their instructors but also their lineage (i.e., where they got their belt). Be wary of anyone who claims to have created their own "fighting system" (only about 1 in every 100,000 of these end up being worthwhile). If a school makes claims on its website that it can turn you into a black belt in a specified period of time, it should be avoided. Schools like that are referred to as "Belt Factories."

Next, go to the school while a class is in session to check it out. First and foremost, it should be clean inside. This doesn't mean shiny and spotless; it is a place of sweat and toil, after all. Simply, it shouldn't smell like an unwashed gym towel, and you shouldn't see fingernails and hairballs on the floor. A dirty martial arts academy is a sign of an instructor who lacks pride and discipline, and that isn't someone you want to learn from. Speaking of the instructor, look at him or her. Having a black belt is great, but having a stomach that protrudes out so far that you cannot even see that belt is another matter. A martial arts instructor should be in good shape—not necessarily on the cover of Men's Health magazine, but if they look like they are more likely to win a hot-dog-eating contest as opposed to a martial arts tournament, that's a red flag. Typically, the instructor or someone else should greet you and ask if you are interested in classes. Be wary of any place that requires you to sign a contract without allowing you to participate in at least a class or two to see how you like it. Watch the class, and see how the instructor interacts with the students. A good instructor should be firm but not domineering, encouraging but not coddling, and should train and spar with the students. I would not even consider studying any martial art that did not include sparring and would not study under any instructor who did not spar with the students.

Now, on to *why* the practice of martial arts is not just great for fitness but highly beneficial to personal development and wellness.

It is my opinion that ego is the enemy of success. Ego allows you to go through life thinking you are invincible while blinding you to your own shortcomings. Ego can get you into dangerous situations and prevents you from seeing things objectively. When someone gets physically injured doing something they shouldn't have, ego is often the culprit. When a company goes from making millions to sudden bankruptcy, it can often be traced to bad decisions in the boardroom that were based on collective corporate ego, centered on the belief that the company could not fail.

Relationships often fail because of ego, whether that is a person's inability to admit when they are at fault or the narcissism that drives infidelity. An inflated ego is perhaps the greatest impediment to personal growth known to man. History is full of the tales of battles and even entire wars lost due to a commander's ego.

Martial arts and BJJ, in particular (in my opinion), deconstruct the ego. There is nothing more humbling than going to class and being choked unconscious by someone 15 years your senior whom you outweigh by 30 pounds (yes, it has happened to me).

I didn't start BJJ until well into my 40s. Although I had "dabbled" in martial arts throughout my life and had trained in Army hand-to-hand combat (which was actually pretty useless until around 2001 when the Army fixed it), I really didn't have any legitimate training in unarmed self-defense. The day I walked into my first BJJ class, I was already a Ranger and a Green Beret who had seen combat. To look at my resume, anyone would think that I was a "certified badass." An experienced BJJ brown belt even once asked me, a white belt at the time, why I felt that I had anything to prove. The answer is simple: we *always* have something to prove, and the best way to do that is by actually *proving it* in the form of testing yourself. On the mats, one on one with an opponent, it makes no difference who has a more impressive list of accomplishments, or who drives a nicer car, or who makes more money. The mat and the sparring ring are like combat in that they are raw and real, exposing what people are made of. You can't fake it when it is real.

If you choose to practice BJJ as I recommend, all the aforementioned guidelines for choosing a school apply. Additionally, I would add that not even BJJ is immune from the "softening" that comes along with wider mainstream exposure. There are BJJ schools that emphasize "sport" BJJ over the traditional fighting style made famous by the Gracie family. If you find yourself in a sport-oriented academy, it isn't the end of the world. Just be aware that some things may work well in competition (where there are rules) but be dangerous to you if used in actual self-defense. You can fill in these gaps with seminars and video tutorials from self-defense experts and by seeking out others in your school or area to train with who have a similar focus toward practical self-defense. Also, do not be timid about (respectfully) asking your instructor about the validity of certain moves and techniques in self-defense scenarios.

Bottom line: choose a martial art and an academy that is practical and allows you to pressure test. In doing so, you will have a realistic understanding of how prepared you *actually* are for a physical altercation. If you are grounded in reality, then you understand the world you live in, and if you understand the world you live in, then you know what your place is in it.

TAKEAWAYS

- The practice of martial arts contributes to all aspects of wellness. (It's like yoga you can defend yourself with.)
- Decide what you want out of martial arts, and pick your style and school accordingly. (Do your research, and beware of frauds.)
- Ego is the enemy of success. (Pressure testing yourself in martial arts deconstructs the ego.)
- Martial arts provides an *objective* assessment of your fitness. (The mirror might lie to you, but the mat will not.)
- Brazilian Jiu Jitsu is the way to go. (You don't have to take my word for it, but you should.)

✳ CHAPTER 7 ✳

RECOVERY

How we recover and how often we recover is of equal importance to how we workout, possibly more so. The misconception that most of us were brought up with was that recovery and rest are synonymous—they aren't. *Rest* is inactivity, while *recovery* is the action of returning to a better or more healthy state. This isn't to say that resting is not also a form of recovery; it is. Complete rest is what we refer to as *passive recovery*, whereas *active recovery* is exactly what it sounds like: taking action to aid your body in its recovery.

Active recovery is vital for the elimination of lactic acid, maintaining flexibility/mobility, and keeping you engaged in your fitness regimen both physically and mentally. Walking, swimming, light jogging, yoga, Tai Chi, bike riding, etc. are all forms of active recovery. There are even ways that you can start your active recovery the moment you complete a workout, without waiting for the next day.

Doing a cooldown after a workout is important to "equilibrate" your body, not only so that you aren't walking out of the gym, still breathing hard with your heart pounding, but also to help eliminate byproducts of cellular metabolism and initiate healing during the phase when blood flow to the tissues is maximized. During any workout where you have reached the anaerobic level, especially working power and/or high intensity muscle endurance, your muscle cells produce lactic acid. We have all felt that next-day soreness and stiffness that comes from a combination of lactic-acid buildup and microdamage to our tissues. When muscles burn glycogen for fuel, the byproduct is lactic acid, which is pumped out of the cell and is deposited in the interstitial tissue until the lymphatic system can take it away to be eliminated. Unlike our circulatory system, the lymphatic system does not have a central "pump" to keep everything moving. In order for the lymphatics to move fluid, they require the surrounding tissue to "squeeze" them and push the fluid past a series of valves. If we are sedentary after a workout, the lactic acid remains in our interstitial tissues, and we feel it the next day in the form of soreness. Through activity, we contract the muscles around the lymphatic vessels and provide the necessary "squeeze" to move the fluid along. A 10- to 15-minute cooldown can be highly beneficial in this regard. (There are some other ways to accomplish this with the aid of technology.) Many fitness coaches will advise the use of foam rollers and trigger balls immediately post workout to stretch muscles and fascia as well as facilitate elimination of lactic acid via mechanical assistance in the form of pressure.

If, like me, you elect to devote a specific day on your schedule to active recovery, I recommend one of the aforementioned physical activities. Wear your heart monitor and be mindful of not pushing yourself hard. Remember, this is a recovery, not a workout. Your heart rate shouldn't get any higher than the low threshold of your aerobic zone (if that), and you shouldn't feel overly taxed at any point. A light sweat is a good thing, but a puddle on the floor means you went too far (unless, of course, you are in a hot yoga studio or sauna). Because you are eliminating toxins, your level of hydration should be equal to a regular workout day (very important!). Having a plan for active recovery is *extremely important!* Don't tell yourself you are going to do "something" because then you won't. Designate a specific time and specific activity. I recommend 45 minutes to an hour. If you end up with two scheduled recovery days in a row, make sure to conduct active recovery on the first day, when your body needs it most. This allows you to enjoy your passive recovery day without issue.

For me, even passive recovery involves some planning and action. On those days, I will perform some brief mobility exercises early in the day, for both mental and physical reasons. If I have been noticing issues with my joints or some injuries, I may apply an ice pack to a sore joint and follow up with some passive range of motion exercises. If I am having issues with sore muscles, then a sauna, a soak in a hot tub, or a deep tissue massage is in order.

I have been asked quite a bit about whole-body cryotherapy (WBC) and its benefits. WBC is subjecting your body to extremely cold, dry air, usually in a cabinet that operates using liquid nitrogen. My own personal experience was positive, with my sore joints feeling better and my muscles feeling recharged after the session, but the human studies I have reviewed show no significant difference compared to placebo. Even though I have done it and liked it, I cannot endorse the practice in good conscience unless (or until) scientific evidence comes along showing it is effective. In fact, studies show WBC can significantly hamper the body's anabolic response that occurs after training, which prevents repair and rebuilding and is, therefore, counterproductive.

Something that does have scientific studies to back it up is intermittent pneumatic compression (IPC) performed immediately post-exercise to facilitate lymphatic drainage. As I stated earlier, the lymphatic system is what removes lactic acid from the tissue following anaerobic exercise. I was recently introduced to IPC, which involves placing both legs into a set of inflatable "boots," which cover your legs from foot to thigh and intermittently inflate and deflate to "squeeze" your legs, thereby aiding in lymphatic drainage. After my positive experience, I consulted the literature and was very pleased to see that some solid science exists to back up the practice. If you train somewhere that has this type of device, I highly recommend trying it out, especially after a heavily anaerobic leg workout.

In addition to active and passive recovery as a part of your weekly program, you will also need to consider periods of *de-loading* as your fitness program progresses. Put simply, de-loading is when you have a planned decrease in both the amount of training that you are doing as well as the intensity of that training. De-loading becomes important when your workouts become higher in volume and intensity, as a means to allow adequate musculoskeletal and neurologic recovery. Without de-loading, you risk injury and burnout from over training, as well as reach a point of diminishing returns.

In the early stages of working out, when you aren't pushing the boundaries of your physical performance, de-loading isn't something you need to worry about until around the eighth or even twelfth week of your routine. When you are working out intensely and really engrossed in the high-performance lifestyle of the warrior-athlete, you may need to de-load as often as every four weeks (working out for four weeks and de-loading on the fifth before starting again).

Again, this is an area where a fitness coach or trainer can be invaluable.

The technique that I recommend for de-loading is to simply reduce both weight and repetitions for resistance/weight training while doing the same lifts/exercises or at least the same basic movements (i.e., if you are doing zercher squats, you can change it to goblet squats during your de-load period). Similarly, for endurance exercises, I like to cut back the intensity and the duration, basically keeping out of the anaerobic zone entirely for that week, not even touching it. Everything I do for flexibility and mobility remains mostly the same, and I may add an extra yoga session that week. Likewise, I dial back the intensity of my martial arts training and concentrate on refining my technique above all else. I have found that I feel amazing the week following my de-load, and it really energizes me and keeps me in the game.

Often times, I try and schedule my de-loads for weeks that I otherwise would have to modify my workout anyway. I didn't cover this in the chapter on fitness, but it is a fact of life that we all have those weeks where "life gets in the way," whether it is a business trip, a vacation, or a family commitment that keeps you out of the gym for a week. These unavoidable life events can be an ideal time for a de-load. In a hotel gym, the hotel room itself, in a park, or on your back porch, you can do a scaled-down facsimile of your regular workout. This will provide the necessary de-load, while maintaining mobility, flexibility, and durability, as well as keeping you sharp and focused. Even 30 minutes a day can be enough to get just enough blood flowing to be beneficial while not taxing your system and not eating into your busy schedule. A couple times a year, I have to travel to Israel for business, and every morning, I jog on the beach, swim in the ocean, and do some light dumbbell work. I have done kickboxing pad work in the park in Tel Aviv just to stay sharp and get a sweat going. It also helps with my jet lag and keeps me from gaining travel weight from all that great food.

Be careful to continue to watch your nutrition and hydration during your de-load and be mindful of the fact that you are expending fewer calories, which means you need to be ingesting less. Make sure those reductions are not at the expense of protein, and preferentially reduce your carbohydrates instead. A word of caution: don't turn a de-load into a vacation and allow yourself to over-indulge. Think of de-loading as a *part* of your workout routine, not a break from it.

TAKEAWAYS

- Recovery is vital (equally important to exercise, if not more so).
- Rest can be recovery, but not all recovery is rest. (Active recovery can be even more beneficial.)

- Recovery starts during the workout cooldown. (Don't just stop and walk away when the last repetition is done.)
- Plan exactly what your active and passive recovery days will consist of. (They are as much a part of your fitness routine as your workouts.)
- Schedule "de-load" weeks periodically. (You can't always run the racecar in the red.)
- Adjust your calories/nutrition during recovery, and de-load. (Your body still needs building blocks, but do not overeat when you aren't burning as much fuel.)

✳ CHAPTER 8 ✳

SUPPLEMENTS

Supplements are a topic that comes up quite a bit, and it means different things to different people. Rather than hash out all the definitions that are out there, I will tell you how I define them so that we are on the same page.

I define supplements as any substance taken above and beyond normal foods and beverages for the expressed purpose of providing either macronutrients (protein, carbohydrates, or fats), micronutrients (vitamins and essential minerals/electrolytes), or organic substances/compounds (creatine, amino acids, fish oil, turmeric, etc.). Basically, anything taken other than food to provide health benefits, not including pharmaceuticals.

The supplement business is a multi-billion-dollar industry,

and to be honest, most of what is out there is probably useless. Especially when it comes to vitamin supplements, the debate has raged for decades as to whether or not there is any proven benefit. In truth, most studies have shown that if people eat a healthy and balanced diet, there is probably little to no benefit from taking supplemental vitamins. The gap in these studies is threefold: first, they assume everyone is eating healthy when we know that is not the case; second, they typically have addressed supplements as an umbrella term, not looking at specifics; third, the studies have concentrated on *average* people performing an *average* amount of activity, not performance athletes. (Let's be real, if you are reading this book and have made it this far, you are truly a warrior-athlete and are far from average.)

In the past, I did nothing more than take a multivitamin each day, even though I knew that a lot of what was in it was doing nothing more than changing the color of my urine. It wasn't until I got a little older that I decided to do a deep dive into individual supplements of all categories to see what the science had to say about their effectiveness. I looked not just at vitamins and minerals but at other organic supplements that had been touted to provide health benefits that I felt were relevant to me and needed for my specific health and performance. What I discovered was that there was very solid evidence for some supplements and either no evidence or contradictory evidence for others. I didn't research everything that is out there—I simply do not have that much time—but I did research what I thought to be pertinent, and then incorporated that research accordingly into my personal regimen. What I will share with you in this chapter is what I take, why I take it, and the science behind it.

Let's start with what I take in the morning. I feel it is important to "pre-load" on some things before the day gets going to address deficiencies, before they have a chance to occur, and start the process of proper healing prior to doing a workout.

CURCUMIN

Like most military veterans, I spent a lot of years taking Nonsteroidal Anti-inflammatories (NSAIDs) such as Ibuprofen on virtually a daily basis. As I have said, part of the warrior-athlete lifestyle is a certain degree of both acute and chronic musculoskeletal injuries. But since the mission must continue, many of us developed the habit of taking 800 mg of "Ranger Candy" with breakfast in the morning, just to get enough relief to perform. The long-term side effects of NSAIDs include stomach ulcers, kidney damage, and heart problems, among other things. Like many people, I discovered curcumin as a natural and safer alternative to NSAIDs.

Derived from a plant in the ginger family, multiple research studies suggest that *curcumin* can be of benefit in the management of inflammatory conditions, acute and chronic musculoskeletal pain, and arthritis. There is even evidence to suggest that it can be beneficial in certain metabolic syndromes, alleviate anxiety, and help with hyperlipidemia (elevated cholesterol and/or triglycerides). Curcumin has also been shown to have a positive effect on cognition and mood. I take 500 mg twice a day (morning and night with food) to help prevent and treat muscle and joint pain from working out and from getting beat up in BJJ.

BIOPERINE

Bioperine was something I discovered by accident. In looking at the ingredients in a lot of supplements, I kept seeing it. Out of curiosity, I did some research and discovered its origin and its properties. Bioperine is an extract from the black pepper fruit (also known as "peppercorn"). It is a secondary substance in many supplements because of its ability to boost the bioavailability of a number of therapeutic drugs and phytochemicals (including curcumin). It does this by stimulating the body to release certain digestive enzymes and activating some cellular transport channels. Bioperine has also been found to have independent beneficial health effects, particularly in the realm of diet-induced oxidative stress secondary to consumption of fats. In other words, it is a potent antioxidant. I take 10 mg of bioperine with my curcumin, morning and night, to help with digestion and for its other benefits.

VITAMIN D3

Vitamin D is vital for bone health and immune system function and has been shown to have a positive effect on mood, as well as reduce both chronic and acute pain. In 2008, *The American Journal on Clinical Nutrition* published an article recognizing a global epidemic of vitamin D deficiency. You may have heard vitamin D referred to as the "Sun Vitamin," as cells in our skin have the ability to convert cholesterol into vitamin D. In our youth, most of us didn't have any issue with adequate vitamin D, as we were raised drinking milk and spent plenty of time playing outside. As we have aged and as society has undergone changes that find us spending less time out in the sun, this has become more of an issue. A few years ago, my doctor informed me that my vitamin D levels were low and suggested I take a supplement. Since then, I have added it to my morning and evening regimen. A word of caution: contrary to popular belief, you can take too much when it comes to vitamins, particularly the fat-soluble vitamins, which are A, D, E, and K, as those build up in your system as opposed to being eliminated in your urine. Be mindful of the percentage of the recommended daily allowance (RDA) that you are taking, and consider getting specific guidelines on intake from your doctor based on your laboratory values. I take 2,000 iu (International Units), morning and night.

ZINC

When I was a third-year medical student on my surgical rotation, we had an elderly patient who was not healing well from her surgery. This prompted a two-hour lecture on *zinc* from one of the attending physicians. He described it as, "One of the cheapest, most abundant, and yet absolutely essential trace minerals on the planet." I learned that zinc is vital for healing, proper tissue repair (especially collagen synthesis), and our immune system. Zinc deficiency is what causes stretch marks in pregnant women. Numerous aspects of cellular metabolism are zinc-dependent, and it is a key element in over 100 catalytic enzymes throughout the human body. I take 20 mg of zinc, morning and night, to help with healing and overall health. Be careful not to take too much zinc, as it can indirectly cause a copper deficiency.

VITAMIN C

We grew up hearing about the health benefits of *vitamin C* and were encouraged to drink our orange juice, so we wouldn't get sick. Like zinc, vitamin C is required for wound healing and the biosynthesis of collagen and certain neurotransmitters. It is also involved in protein metabolism and is a physiological antioxidant. It has an important role in immune function and improves iron absorption (vital for hemoglobin production in our red blood cells). I take 50 mg of vitamin C twice a day with my zinc.

FISH OIL

I was a little late to the fish oil "party." I had heard about it but thought it was another fad supplement. It wasn't until a friend of mine, Dr. Andrew Winge, told me about the benefits of taking a fish-oil supplement that I took an interest. The long-chain omega-3 fatty acids found in fish oil are eicosapentaenoic acid (EPA) and docosahexaenoic acid (DHA). Omega-3 fatty acids are an integral part of cell membranes throughout the body and influence the function of the cell receptors in these membranes. They are important in brain health and the regulation of inflammatory response. They also bind to receptors in cells that regulate genetic function. Omega-3 fats have been shown to help prevent heart disease and stroke and may be beneficial in alleviating a variety of adverse health conditions including arthritis and some forms of cancer. You may also be familiar with *krill oil*, which has a lot of the same properties as fish oil, but some studies have shown it to be even more potent. Krill oil is a great alternative and, arguably, may even be better, but it is a little more expensive and can be harder to find. As long as you are getting EPA and DHA from clean and organic sources, you should be good to go in this department. Whichever I am taking, whether it is fish oil or krill oil, I take it twice a day. It is usually found in softgels, but you can also find it in flavored liquid and creme forms that can be taken alone or added to coffee, which some people prefer. I currently take 1,000 mg of omega-3 fish oil twice daily.

CORDYCEPS MUSHROOM EXTRACT

I first heard about *Cordyceps mushroom extract* while listening to the Joe Rogan podcast. The Cordyceps sinensis mushroom has been used in traditional Chinese medicine for centuries and is considered a natural energy booster. Proponents also claim that Cordyceps can protect against health problems like asthma, depression, diabetes, fatigue, and high cholesterol, as well as boost both athletic performance and male sexual function. What I found through research was that there is a ton of data showing that Cordyceps can be helpful for performance athletes and that it improves oxygen utilization at the cellular level, particularly during low-oxygen states such as high altitude. I bought some and started taking it before BJJ class. I found that my exercise tolerance and stamina were immediately and noticeably improved. This is another twice-a-day supplement for me, either at breakfast and dinner or timed 30 minutes before my workouts/training sessions. I have found that taking 300 mg twice a day yields excellent results.

ACETYL-L-CARNITINE

Much like bioperine, *acetyl-L-carnitine* was an ingredient that I kept seeing in other supplements, so I looked further into it. Acetyl-L-carnitine is a form of *L-carnitine*, which is an amino acid found in nearly all the cells of the body. As I am sure you know, amino acids are the building blocks of proteins. L-carnitine plays a critical role in the production of energy from long-chain fatty acids, and it increases the activity of certain nerve cells in the central nervous system. Acetyl-L-carnitine is used as a supplement to improve memory and cognition and alleviate chronic pain and symptoms of depression. It has also been studied for its potential to help in male and female infertility. I take 300 mg twice a day to help with focus and cognition. I have found that I feel more mentally sharp when I am taking it.

RESVERATROL

For decades, I had heard anecdotal reports of the health and longevity benefits of red wine. Although I never considered myself to be a red wine aficionado (my wife is, however), I was interested in the clinical validity of these claims. What I discovered through research was that *resveratrol*, a substance found in the skin of wine grapes, has been determined to be the source of these benefits. Studies have shown that resveratrol can improve insulin resistance and lipid metabolism throughout the body. It is a potent antioxidant that protects cells from damage secondary to free radicals. This is important, as it is believed to provide a significant benefit to cardiovascular health. There is also some evidence that resveratrol may improve mitochondrial function (the portion of our cells that produce energy). You may recall from earlier in the book that resveratrol may also boost the function of adenosine monophosphate-activated protein kinase (AMPK), which is integral for cellular health throughout the human body. I supplement resveratrol with a 300-mg dose twice daily, and I am also more likely to have a glass of red wine than I used to be.

L-CITRULLINE

A few years ago, a patient presented to my ER for a shoulder dislocation, which had occurred while he was competing in a handstand pushup contest. The patient was five years older than I was at the time and appeared to be the picture of health (other than the shoulder dislocation). As is standard procedure, he was asked to list all medications he was currently taking, which included a prescription for seasonal allergies and a list of natural supplements. I recognized all the supplements on the list except for *L-Citrulline*, so I asked him about it. He told me that he took it as a natural alternative to blood-pressure medication and as a form of "natural Viagra." His blood pressure in the ER was great, even with the pain of his shoulder, and although I didn't ask about the Viagra effect, he and his lovely wife certainly appeared to have a great relationship. I made a note and did some research on my next day off, discovering some interesting things. L-citrulline is a *non-essential* amino acid. Your kidneys change L-citrulline into the *essential* amino acid *L-arginine* and a chemical called *nitric oxide*. These compounds are important to your heart and blood vessel health and may also boost your immune system.

Nitric oxide helps your arteries relax and work more efficiently, which improves blood flow throughout your body. (This is the same mechanism of action of Viagra and other erectile-dysfunction medications.) There is some evidence to suggest the supplement could possibly help lower blood pressure in people with prehypertension, boost athletic performance, and improve male sexual performance. I currently take 600 mg twice a day as part of what I refer to as my "vitality" regimen.

I don't like the term "pre-workout" because it covers such a broad range of supplements, many of which are overly high in both caffeine and sugar. The one or two times in my youth I took a pre-workout, I felt such a "jolt" that I was actually concerned my heart rate might get too high. As I have gotten older, I have come to see the value in a natural boost of energy before a workout or at key points in the day when you might need a little extra energy to get you going. What I am going to discuss next are some of the supplements I have found to have good data as far as both safety and efficacy when it comes to energy boosting.

TAURINE

Found in many energy drinks and pre-workout formulations, *taurine* is an amino acid found naturally in meat, fish, and dairy products. It crosses the blood-brain barrier and is one of the most abundant amino acids in the brain and spinal cord. Taurine is essential for cardiovascular health and development and the normal function of skeletal muscle. It is also essential to the function of the central nervous system, including the formation and maintenance of the retina of the eye. This is extremely important, as there are a litany of retinal problems that can develop with age. Studies suggest that taurine supplementation may improve athletic performance and mental focus, either alone or in combination with other dietary supplements. At least one study showed that vegans have a propensity to taurine deficiency, as it is only found in animal products. I take 1,000 mg to give me a mental and physiological boost, either early in the day or 30 minutes before a workout.

L-THEANINE

I am not sure how I first heard about *L-theanine*, but I believe it was as one of the active ingredients in green tea back when that beverage first gained widespread popularity. It is an *essential* amino acid that elevates levels of neurotransmitters such as serotonin, dopamine, and Gamma aminobutyric acid (GABA). These neurotransmitters work in the brain to regulate emotions, mood, concentration, alertness, appetite, energy, and some higher cognitive skills. By itself, it has something of a calming effect and reduces anxiety, but with caffeine it has the synergistic effect of providing focus and alertness, without the anxious feeling that accompanies many stimulants. I find that adding 100 mg of L-theanine to my "energy" formula makes me feel sharp and also lifts my mood.

NIACIN (VITAMIN B3)

In medical school, I learned about a condition known as *pellagra*, which is niacin deficiency. Initially manifested by gastrointestinal and skin symptoms, it can progress to severe neurological impairment. *Niacin* is an extremely important micronutrient. In fact, every part of your body needs it to function properly. As a supplement, niacin may help lower cholesterol, ease arthritis, and boost brain function. When I saw that it was present in a lot of pre-workout and energy formulations I was curious as to why. What I found through both research and personal experience was that niacin provides a neurological "boost" without a subsequent "crash." Fifteen milligrams of niacin is an integral part of my energy regimen.

PYRIDOXINE HCL (VITAMIN B6)

Vitamin B6 in coenzyme form performs a wide variety of functions in the body and is extremely versatile, with involvement in more than 100 enzyme reactions, mostly pertaining to protein metabolism. Vitamin B6 also plays a role in cognitive development through the synthesis of neurotransmitters and by maintaining normal levels of homocysteine (an amino acid). High levels of homocysteine are associated with heart disease, so both B6 and B12 are vital to keep it in check. Vitamin B6 is involved in gluconeogenesis and glycogenolysis, immune function, and hemoglobin formation. B6 is in the trio of B vitamins I use as energy boosters, along with B3 (discussed), and B12 (up next). I find taking 2 mg to be sufficient.

COBALAMIN (VITAMIN B12)

Vitamin B12 is involved in the metabolism and function of every cell of the human body and plays a vital role in the maturation of developing red blood cells in the bone marrow. It is a cofactor in DNA synthesis as well as both fatty acid and amino acid metabolism. It is particularly important in the normal functioning of the nervous system due to its role in myelin synthesis. B12 deficiency goes hand in hand with anemia and neurological disorders. 2.5 mcg of B12 is a vital part of my B-vitamin energy trio.

YERBA MATE

While I was in the 7th Special Forces Group (Airborne), our area of operations was Central and South America. During that time, on one of my numerous deployments, I was introduced to *yerba mate*, which many South Americans drink as a tea. Yerba mate comes from the naturally caffeinated leaves of *Ilex Paraguariensis*, a native holly tree found deep in the South American rainforest. It contains

24 vitamins and minerals, 15 amino acids, and multiple polyphenols (plant-based micronutrients). Yerba mate is marketed for its reported ability to suppress appetite and burn fat, and some studies show that it can help reverse the adverse health effects associated with obesity. Yerba mate has potent anti-inflammatory and antioxidant properties. A study showed that subjects taking yerba mate were able to reduce their LDL cholesterol within 20 days of supplementation. It is also believed to protect the heart and cardiovascular system. I have found it to be a natural and efficient way to get a caffeine boost by taking 300 mg when I need it.

Another important consideration when thinking about both pre- and post-workout is *substrate*, or fuel. In addition to all the "boosting" supplements that I described, you need to have fuel to burn, which is all about nutrition. Supplementation isn't an excuse to have poor nutrition. Post workout, your body is going to require both replacement fuel and the raw materials to build and repair. Now, I would like to address a couple of key supplements post workout.

CREATINE

Creatine has been well known and highly used in the world of fitness for some time, with a lot of debate on whether or not supplementation was safe and effective (it is). Creatine is an amino acid found in all of your skeletal muscles. It helps recycle and replenish *adenosine triphosphate (ATP)*, which is the fuel we burn at the cellular level. Studies have shown that creatine supplementation helps improve muscle power, in that it is key during short bursts of muscle contraction of less than three minutes in duration. I have found that if I do not take creatine after my workout early in the day, I struggle with BJJ sparring that evening, as my muscles cannot recycle ATP as efficiently. I mix 5 g of creatine with my protein supplement and take it immediately post workout.

PROTEIN

As I have already talked about protein and how much we require, I won't belabor the point here. What I do want to address is the fact that your body requires protein within a relatively short window after workout (*how* short is the topic of much debate). As far as the *source* of that protein, I recommend whey. Whey is a dairy product isolated during the cheese-making process. Most importantly, it is a *complete* protein, which means it contains adequate portions of the nine *essential* amino acids (the amino acids your body cannot produce on its own). Although there are some plant proteins that are also complete, they typically take longer to digest and become bioavailable for use (nutritionists recommend that those using plant protein supplements ingest them *prior* to working out instead of afterwards for this very reason). The debate on animal protein vs. plant protein fills entire books in itself, so I am not going down that rabbit hole in depth. Suffice it to say that I personally choose grass-fed whey protein, and I take 20 g in the form of a shake within 30 minutes post workout. I also eat a banana with the shake for two reasons: the carbohydrates in the banana will cause a slight rise in insulin levels, which facilitates transport of both protein and creatine into my cells, and it helps replace any muscle glycogen that I burned during my workout.

As I illustrated earlier, there are certain supplements that I take twice a day, while others (those with stimulants) are reserved for only early in the day. You may recall from the chapter on sleep that I covered nighttime sleep supplements in depth, so there is no reason to rehash that list in detail here.

This last supplement I think bears mentioning: *cannabidiol (CBD)*. CBD is an extract derived from the cannabis plant that has become increasingly popular in recent years with many theories and claims as to its benefits. Although not the panacea that some have made it out to be, it has been shown to be beneficial for certain uses.

CBD has shown clear benefits in the treatment of anxiety, insomnia, and chronic pain. Having taken it myself, I can personally attest to its value, especially in aiding in restful sleep. For those times when I have early-morning commitments, have changed time zones, or am experiencing some added stress, I have found CBD tincture to be a preferable alternative to prescription sleep aids. I use it sparingly, as my normal regimen of natural sleep supplements is usually sufficient.

I am closely watching the data on CBD as it becomes available, as I think it is certainly something promising. Whether or not it is right for you depends on a lot of factors, including the fact that you may be subject to urinalysis because of your vocation. There are varying levels of *tetrahydrocannabinol (THC)*, the active ingredient in marijuana, in CBD. If you take a CBD formulation that is "hot," it is possible to test positive on a drug test. For this reason, many organizations, including the US Military, do not allow their personnel to take CBD products. This is a "consult your doctor" situation. You should also consult your boss and pay careful attention to where you are getting your CBD and how tightly it is quality controlled.

The "consult your doctor" advice applies to any and all supplements but especially if you are already taking prescription medications, as there can be serious interactions. Although monitored for safety, supplements are not stringently regulated by the Food and Drug Administration (FDA) and, therefore, can be tricky to navigate. I encourage you to look at the supplements I have researched and decide what might be right for you based on your own needs. My list, and this chapter, are by no means an all-inclusive list of what is out there that has potential benefit. Much like exercise and diet, see what works for you, and research any claims that you happen to come across. That is what I have done and continue to do, and I am always looking to update and improve what I take on a daily basis.

TAKEAWAYS

- Consult your doctor before starting any supplements. (They can interact with medications, and some supplements shouldn't be taken by certain people.)
- What I *currently* take is as follows (your particular supplements and dosages may vary):
- Morning:
  - Longevity formula:
    - Curcumin: 500 mg
    - Bioperine: 10 mg
    - Vitamin D3: 2,000 iu
    - Zinc: 20 mg
    - Vitamin C: 50 mg
    - Omega-3 fish oil: 1,000 mg
  - Vitality formula:
    - Cordyceps mushroom extract: 300 mg
    - Acetyl-L-carnitine: 300 mg
    - Resveratrol: 300 mg
    - L-citrulline: 600 mg
- Pre-workout:

- Energy formula:
  - Taurine: 1,000 mg
  - L-theanine: 100 mg
  - Niacin: 15 mg
  - Vitamin B6: 2 mg
  - Vitamin B12: 2.5 mcg
  - Yerba mate: 300 mg
- Post-workout:
  - Whey protein: 20 g
  - Creatine: 5 g
- Evening:
  - Longevity formula:
    - Curcumin: 500 mg
    - Bioperine: 10 mg
    - Vitamin D3: 2,000 iu
    - Zinc: 20 mg
    - Vitamin C: 50 mg
    - Omega-3 fish oil: 1,000 mg
  - Vitality formula:
    - Cordyceps mushroom extract: 300 mg
    - Acetyl-L-carnitine: 300 mg
    - Resveratrol: 300 mg
    - L-citrulline: 600 mg
  - Sleep formula (as needed):
    - Melatonin: 3 mg
    - Magnesium: 400 mg
    - Valerian root: 400 mg
    - L-tryptophan: 650 mg

- Look for clinical evidence when evaluating if a supplement is right for you. (There's a lot out there that does nothing and is just a waste of money.)

✳ CHAPTER 9 ✳

HEALTH MAINTENANCE

One of the biggest holes in the American healthcare system is *preventive medicine*: how we approach treating illness by avoiding it in the first place through patient education and health maintenance. The fact that we do such a poor job has fed into the myth that "the medical community wants people to get sick because healthcare is a business." That statement is not only naive but patently untrue. It has been picked up as a clarion call by everyone from small-time snake-oil hucksters with fake cures to those who seek to destroy our system and install one that they can more readily control and profit from.

The fact of the matter is we are impatient as a society and have a lot on our plate as individuals, so the majority of people don't even want to think about their health until something goes wrong and they need medical attention. As I have stated before, the medical community has done a great disservice in enabling this behavior by holding up "cures" as a free ticket for people to ignore their health until the last possible minute, then come running to us for pills, treatments, or surgeries. The fact that you have waded your way through this far into my haranguing tells me that you aren't like that at all. You're willing to put in the work in advance, even though you may have already kicked that can down the road for a few decades already. So, let's remedy that problem on a personal level and start addressing it now. In addition to eating a proper diet, exercising, not smoking, and drinking alcohol only in moderation, there are certain things you should do to keep ahead of your health. Like I tell my patients, take *ownership* of your health, and don't leave it in anyone else's hands. Nobody is going to care about you and your health as much as you do, and nobody else knows more about you and your body.

I already touched on this topic in the chapter on aging. In this chapter, I will reiterate and go into more depth as to what you should be doing to address health screening and maintenance.

ROUTINE PHYSICAL EXAMS

Starting at age 40, you should have a routine doctor's appointment and examination every other year even if you have no chronic issues and aren't on any medications. Obviously, anyone on prescription medications or being followed for any condition should be seen more frequently. Once you reach age 50, the frequency should change to once per year. There is specific laboratory work that should be checked, which I will cover under the appropriate sections further ahead.

CARDIOVASCULAR SCREENING

If you don't have significant risk for cardiovascular disease (smoking, obesity, diabetes, high blood pressure, significant family history, etc.), then routine screening is fairly straightforward.

At age 40, a blood pressure check becomes an important part of the routine screening process. If you don't have any issues, then every two years is typically fine. Unless your doctor specifically prescribes a home blood pressure machine and gives you specific instructions as to how often and when to check it, do not buy one. Home blood pressure machines are notoriously inaccurate and probably cause tens of thousands of unnecessary medical visits for every potential medical problem they identify.

Cholesterol screening is important in determining your risk for heart attack and stroke. Expect your doctor to check your LDL and HDL cholesterol and your triglycerides every two years at age 40 and probably every year at age 50. If an abnormality is detected, then screening will be more frequent. Likewise, a check of your fasting blood sugar to determine if you are diabetic or pre-diabetic is an important screening tool. Family history or obesity could dictate that these values require regular monitoring at an even earlier age.

Stepping on the scale to get your weight is always part of a full physical exam, but it becomes even more important after age 40 in determining your risks for cardiovascular disease. Also expect for them to measure your height, so they can accurately compute your *Body Mass Index (BMI)*. The BMI computation determines how appropriate your weight is in relation to your height. A BMI of less than 18.5 is considered underweight. BMI between 18.5 and 25 is considered normal, while 25–30 is considered overweight and above 30 is classified as obese. The average BMI for an adult male in the United States is 26.6 (overweight), according to the CDC. If you would like to know your BMI, there are multiple online BMI calculators you can use, and some "smart scales" will do it for you.

Note: as you can see, the "average" BMI and the "normal" BMI are not the same. Never assume that because something is "the average" that it is somehow normal. Allowing people to confuse these terms, using that as an excuse to tolerate the epidemic of obesity in the world today, is another failure of modern medicine.

Your doctor may or may not choose to perform an electro-cardiogram (EKG). Although there is some debate in the medical community as to whether or not screening EKGs should be performed on those with no risk factors, I consider it to be a simple and non-invasive test that establishes what your cardiac activity looks like "at baseline." Ask your doctor if you are a candidate for a *Coronary Calcium Scan (CCS)*. A CCS is used to evaluate how much calcified plaque exists in your coronary arteries and utilizes a scoring system to determine your risk for a cardiac event.

GI SCREENING

As I said in the chapter on aging, screening for colon/col-orectal cancer is something to take seriously. A colonoscopy is recommended every 10 years, starting at age 45, for everyone. For anyone with a first-degree relative with a history of colon cancer (parents or siblings), screening should begin at age 40 (or 10 years prior to the age the family member was diagnosed, whichever comes first). In recent years, non-invasive stool DNA tests have been introduced as an early-screening tool. There are also "virtual colonoscopy" options that can be performed via non-invasive imaging. At age 40, start asking your doctor about which test is right for you and how often you need it.

If you have a history of reflux or other upper gastrointestinal issues, your doctor may perform a screening lab for *Helico-*

bacter Pylori, the bacteria linked to gastric ulcers. You may even be recommended for an upper GI scope if symptoms are chronic or severe.

Laboratory screening to check the function of your liver and gallbladder are a standard part of the chemistry panel your doctor will order during any routine physical. If you are at risk, you may get a hepatitis screening as well.

ENDOCRINE SCREENING

I have already mentioned blood glucose, but it bears repeating as it can be an indication of both impaired pancreatic function and insulin resistance.

Calcium, a normal part of a serum chemistry, can also be a surrogate test for parathyroid hormone function.

Thyroid function should be checked at each visit, especially if you have unexplained weight changes, temperature intolerance, or other issues that could indicate an abnormality. I consider laboratory thyroid tests to be a starting point for many medical workups, especially in older patients.

Not everyone needs their testosterone levels checked, but if you are having issues with energy, libido, exercise tolerance, etc., then a check of both your total testosterone and free testosterone is in order. Most primary care physicians do not have the training to manage low testosterone, so don't be surprised if yours refers you to a specialist, and don't be afraid to insist on seeing someone else if you feel your doctor is out of his or her depth in this area.

SKIN SCREENING

Even during a routine physical exam prior to age 40, your doctor should perform a *total body skin examination (TBSE)*. If you have any lesions at all (moles, skin tags, etc.), I recommend a referral to a dermatologist. No later than age 40, you should be getting a skin cancer screening every year. Those determined by a dermatologist to be of lower risk can probably go every two years, but that determination should be made individually and by a professional. The earlier in your life you begin this process, the better, as the majority of people have at least a few "concerning" lesions by the time they reach middle age. Skin cancer is highly treatable if caught early.

GENITOURINARY SCREENING

Providing a urine sample is a normal part of any complete physical exam, as is a serum chemistry. The two lab tests combined tell your doctor a lot about your kidney function as well as provide other valuable health information. If you have a family history of prostate cancer, you should discuss screening with your doctor as soon as possible. If not, then you should have a discussion with him or her at age 55 pertaining to the risks and benefits of a screening *prostate-specific antigen (PSA)*. This is a change from the previous practice of a digital rectal prostate exam every visit. Unfortunately, testicular/scrotal exams are an uncomfortable but necessary part of a complete physical exam to evaluate both testicular health and check for possible hernias.

MUSCULOSKELETAL SCREENING

There's nothing particularly earth-shattering that your physician will look for when it comes to musculature, although they will evaluate for symmetry and muscle wasting. Bone density scans are not routinely indicated for men, as we are less likely to suffer from osteoporosis. However, if you break a bone while engaged in normal activity (not something that would normally be associated with a broken bone), or if you lose ½ an inch of height in a year, then you would be considered in the higher risk category and should get a scan. Your doctor should be checking your vitamin D levels as soon as you hit age 40 for two reasons: 1) By the time osteoporosis does occur, you are probably ten years behind. 2) Vitamin D deficiency is increasingly common in the western world, and there's really no reason not to check it.

NEUROLOGICAL SCREENING

In addition to checking your reflexes and your *gait* (how

you walk), your doctor should also check your balance and your fine motor skills. This will feel somewhat like a field sobriety test. They should also perform what is known as a *mini mental status exam (MMSE)* to evaluate your short- and long-term memory. If you have a family history of dementia or feel that you may be becoming forgetful, these are things that your doctor needs to know, so they can take them into consideration and adjust their screening exam accordingly.

EYESIGHT SCREENING

Starting at age 40, I recommend an eye exam every year, unless your doctor tells you otherwise. In addition to the standard evaluation of your eyesight, the ophthalmologist or optometrist should also check your visual fields and conduct a glaucoma screening test (usually the puff of air but may consist of numbing drops and a pressure sensor touching your eye). They will examine you for cataracts and will dilate your eyes to visualize the retina and look for any abnormalities. You should also be given an exam known as *Optical Coherence Tomography (OCT)*, which evaluates for macular degeneration. As with anything, let them know about any family history or personal vision changes.

DENTAL

I am terrible about this. Unfortunately, our collective psyche has really connected a lot of negativity with going to the dentist. In addition to brushing, flossing, water picking, etc., you need to get a comprehensive dental exam annually and need to have your teeth professionally cleaned every six months. Remember when we were kids and every adult over 60 seemed to have false teeth? Well, it doesn't have to be that way, but you need to be taking care of your teeth from as young an age as possible.

VACCINATIONS

If you are an anti-vaccine person, then I don't know what to tell you other than I am surprised you have lived long enough to make it this far into the book. I have written and spoken about vaccines and why they are important, and I am not going to rehash it now. Suffice it to say that I firmly believe, based on the science, that you should get vaccinated and should vaccinate your children. Now, let's talk about what vaccines you need as you get older.

In your 40s, unless you work in healthcare or travel places where things like plague and yellow fever are a concern, then you really only need an annual flu vaccine and to keep your tetanus current. FYI: tetanus is a horrendous way to die; I do not recommend it. Make sure you get a tetanus shot every ten years throughout your life.

Starting at age 50, in addition to flu and tetanus, you should also be getting the shingles vaccine. Remember when you were a kid and had chicken pox? Well, guess what: you still have it. The varicella virus has remained dormant in the dorsal root ganglia of your spinal cord all this time like a viral "sleeper agent" just waiting to be activated. If the virus reactivates ("re-animates" sounds cooler, but it isn't as accurate), then you will have an outbreak of blisters along the rib(s) on one side of your body. It can be exquisitely painful and can also lead to a secondary bacterial infection in some cases. Get the shingles vaccine!

In your 60s, it's time to start getting pneumococcal vaccine. You may require this sooner if you have COPD or immune system issues. Ask your doctor.

I made this list as comprehensive as I could, but new recommendations come out each year, and everyone is different. Most important is to see your doctor as often as I indicated as a *minimum* and take your cues from them on what you should be doing and how often. Had I written this chapter two years ago, the recommendations would have been quite different. I have no doubt that two years from now, they will change again. *Discuss age-related medical screening tests with your doctor at each visit!*

TAKEAWAYS

· Take ownership of your health. (Nobody cares about you as much as you do.)

- At age 40, perform minimum screening/maintenance (for those with no health problems):
  - Annual eye exam.
  - Annual dental exam (professional cleaning every six months).
  - Annual skin cancer screening.
  - Annual flu shot.
  - Up-to-date vaccinations including tetanus.
  - Complete physical exam every two years.
    - Vital signs (pulse, respiration, blood pressure, etc.), height and weight, and complete head-to-toe exam.
    - Labs: urinalysis, complete blood count, blood sugar, chemistry to include liver and kidney function, cholesterol, and thyroid function (additional labs performed based on individual history and symptoms).
    - Discuss family history and individual risk factors with your doctor.
    - Consider EKG, Coronary Calcium Score, and specific cancer screenings based on risk factors.
- Colonoscopy/colon cancer screening every ten years beginning at age 45 (sooner if risk factors dictate).
- At age 50, all age 40 requirements continue. Additional requirements as follows (minimum screening/maintenance for those with no health problems):
  - Annual shingles vaccination.

- Change complete physical exam to *annually* (same physical exam requirements as at age 40).
- Add prostate-specific antigen (PSA) blood test to your basic labs at age 55 (adjust based on risk factors).
- At age 60 and beyond, all requirements continue. Discuss additional tests/requirements with your doctor, like including the pneumonia vaccine.

✳ CHAPTER 10 ✳

YOUR TRIBE

I once heard someone say, "There are three types of friends: for a *reason*, for a *season*, and for a *lifetime*." Friends for a *reason* means friends that you make related to a specific activity. They might be your work friends, or your motorcycle friends, or your gym friends. Friends for a *season* are those you associate with during the time that life happens to put you together. This could mean those you went to school with or someone who moves in next door to you. Friends for a *lifetime* are those you have a real connection with because of a shared set of values.

Before I get into the specifics of what I mean by your *tribe* and how it ties into your shared values, let me first give a little background on motivation and discipline that helps illustrate why a tribe is so important.

Motivation is a term you have undoubtedly heard before. I am often asked about how a person can maintain motivation as it applies to working out and being consistent. What I tell people is that motivation is great, but sooner or later, it will wane. What keeps you going isn't motivation; it is *discipline*. Discipline is what gets you to the gym on the days you don't feel like it. Discipline is what pushes you away from the dinner table instead of grabbing an extra helping of mashed potatoes or ordering dessert. When motivation fails, discipline is what keeps you going. Discipline is what makes you do the right thing even when nobody is watching. But what about when both motivation and discipline are running low? What then?

We tend to think of motivation as only coming from within, but that isn't quite true. In addition to *internal* motivation which comes entirely from self, there is also *external* motivation. External motivation can take many different forms, from a drill instructor yelling at you to climb a rope to the threat of death from AK-47 fire motivating you to run for cover. It can also take the form of a goal that you strive to achieve, which could mean an award, praise, or returning home from combat to be reunited with your family. External motivation can be even more powerful than either internal motivation or self-discipline.

Peer pressure (and by that, I mean *positive* peer pressure) can be an extremely helpful form of external motivation. A tribe can provide that.

"You are who you surround yourself with" is a phrase I am sure you have heard. Making positive, long-term lifestyle changes is a lot easier to do if you are surrounded by like-minded people. Your tribe should be made up of people who lift you up and provide positive reinforcement (i.e., motivation) relating to wellness behaviors.

You need to ask yourself a hard question: *are the people in my life lifting me up, or are they holding me back?* Unselfish people should support you in any endeavor that leads to self-improvement and should discourage you from heading down a path to self-destruction. They should celebrate your victories and console you in defeat, while not letting you either rest on your laurels nor wallow in self-pity. I am not saying that every one of your acquaintances has to be going to the gym with you every day, but they also shouldn't be putting obstacles in your path either.

In our age group, it's easy to find BBQ friends, drinking friends, fishing friends, etc. There's no challenge to finding others willing to be *comfortable* with you. What's difficult is finding people willing to be *uncomfortable* with you. The former group are *friends*, while the latter is a *tribe*.

A tribe is about strength, and that strength is only as great as its weakest member. For that reason, the tribe will always strive to bring each individual up to his or her highest possible level. Unlike a circle of friends that is more concerned about what they get back from the group as individuals, the tribe is more about a feeling of community centered on a philosophy. If you've made it this far into this book, then you are at least considering living a life based on a philosophy of health, wellness, and continued self-improvement. To stay on that path, you are going to need to find a tribe that is living that same philosophy. You may not need it in the immediate future, but eventually, you are going to need support and encouragement at a pivotal time, and that is when the tribe will be there to give you that push you need.

A tribe is about accountability, which is why I have found it invaluable. Hey, maybe you aren't like me, and you don't need any external motivation or help. If that's the case, I envy your situation, and you can disregard. But it has been my experience that even the most highly disciplined individuals occasionally need a boost, whether in the form of a pat on the back or a kick in the ass. If it is pride that prevents you from seeking out a support network, then you need to check that at the door right now. The good news is, in this day and age, the tribe doesn't have to be in your immediate geographic area or even be made up of people you know in real life. There are multiple online forums, both on and off social media, that provide this kind of support. Almost all gym memberships and home-exercise plans come with some type of "network" where you can share ideas and get the support and advice of others. But, as I said, the main benefit isn't the guidance; it's the accountability.

I work out alone for the most part, and I like it that way. There have been times when I have had a "gym buddy" to go to the gym with, but other than spotting each other during heavy sets, the majority of the benefit stemmed from the accountability aspect of knowing someone was going to the gym that day and that if I didn't go, I would have to face them and tell them why. Also, a little external motivation in the form of a "C'mon! You've got this!" when that last repetition gets difficult. Now that I work out alone, preferring to have the gym to myself, I don't have that person in real time that I am accountable to. So, there are two ways that I stay accountable to my tribe. First, I use a heart monitor that connects to an app on my phone that all my like-minded friends also have. We can see each other's workouts, and we all know if someone is slacking off. If I go three or four days without logging a workout, I get that, "Hey, man, everything okay?" text message. That's a polite way of asking, "Why aren't you working out? Hurt? Lazy? What's up?" Another way that I stay accountable is by doing "challenges" and special WODs where I get together with like-minded individuals for some camaraderie and motivation. I find once a month to be about right for something like this, so I have to get out there and perform in a group, probably doing exercises that I typically don't do. It keeps me honest, gives me a goal to shoot for, and breaks the monotony. I typically come away from those sessions with a renewed sense of internal motivation and some new ideas on what to incorporate into my regular routine.

My Brazilian Jiu Jitsu tribe has been *instrumental* in keeping me accountable and pushing me to improve. There's nothing more humbling than to miss a few classes and then get choked out by a lower belt who has been putting in the extra practice. I know I said you only compete against yourself, but seeing others improve while you are standing still (ability wise) is a potent wakeup call and motivator. To be a productive member of a martial arts tribe, you should constantly strive for improvement, becoming a better training partner/opponent to the other members of the tribe. If you aren't improving, you aren't just cheating yourself, you're cheating everyone you train with by not being as good as you can be. Someone once asked me what the best way to get better at martial arts was, and I told them, "If you are the toughest person among your friends, then you need to find tougher friends." That sounds harsh, but I meant it, and it is true. Iron sharpens iron.

Bottom line: I am not telling you that you have to abandon everyone in your life who doesn't eat right, workout, and train in martial arts. I am simply saying that anyone who presents an obstacle to you participating in those behaviors is a liability who is holding you back from reaching your full potential, and anyone who supports and motivates you in achieving goals in that arena is an asset. Whether it is a close-knit in-person circle of friends, a social media group of individuals who cheer you on, or some faceless names on a smartphone app who give your workout a thumbs up or a "like," finding that tribe of accountability will reap dividends down the road. Over time, people who have been in your life for years may also want to join this new tribe, as they see the change in you and how positively it has affected all aspects of your life. Just as failure is contagious, so is success. Join a tribe or start your own, share ideas, support one another, and when you reach the mountain top, it will be all that much sweeter because someone is always there to share in the joy of your accomplishment.

TAKEAWAYS

- Seek out relationships based on shared values/philosophy.
- Discipline trumps motivation, but even discipline can be fleeting.
- When internal motivation fails, external motivation can be helpful.
- A tribe is only as strong as its weakest member.
- Being the best version of yourself helps you, other members of the tribe, and the tribe as a whole.
- Find a tribe that will keep you accountable.
- If you are the toughest among your friends, find tougher friends.
- You are who you surround yourself with.

CONCLUSION

LIVE LIFE LIKE A WARRIOR

In the first chapter, I talked about what the definition of a warrior is and how that applies to you living as a warrior-athlete. I hope that through the course of this book you have dog-eared pages, highlighted, underlined, and written notes in the margins. Simply reading these pages in one pass isn't going to set you up for success. It is going to take continuous learning and reinforcement. The best way that you can truly put the ideas in this book into practice is to make the commitment to lifestyle firmly grounded in the warrior ethos. If you get up each and every day and see a warrior looking back at you in the mirror, you will find putting the philosophy of this book into practice all that much easier. If you look at every action throughout your day within the framework of the warrior ethos and ask yourself whether or not what you are doing is beneficial to you as a warrior, you will find that complex decisions become simple. This is especially true as we join the ranks of the "Greybeards," who maintain the warrior lifestyle into the second half of life. Here is why:

One behavior that is never associated with the warrior ethos is resting on one's laurels. Remember when I talked about how, early in my BJJ journey, somebody asked me what I had to prove? Simply put, a warrior *always* has something to prove—not to anyone else but to himself. It is for this reason more than any other that a warrior can live a longer and more fruitful life than those who do not share his ethos. The moment you stop proving to yourself what you are capable of, you start to die a day at a time.

My last team assignment before attending medical school was working as the Intelligence sergeant on a Military Free Fall (MFF or "HALO") team. We had one more deployment to South America scheduled prior to my scheduled release to attend medical school, and the command offered me the opportunity to skip the deployment and stay at home to get ready for my commission and my geographical move. I declined. As a warrior, my place was with my team, especially knowing that on that particular deployment we would be undergoing a rigorous two-week evaluation in a jungle environment. The evaluation would consist of long foot movements through the dense rain forest, navigating rivers in inflatable boats, and crossing mountain ranges on horseback, day and night, over grueling terrain with tactical and survival tasks performed along the way (basically, the military version of an "eco-challenge") There was no way I was going to miss out on such an amazing opportunity to challenge myself.

During that deployment, the 7th Special Forces Group commander came to watch us train. At one point, he pulled me off to the side. He had heard of my upcoming commission and acceptance into medical school and wanted to congratulate me. He asked if everything was going smoothly in the administrative process and if there was anything he could do to facilitate things. We made some small talk, and he jokingly asked me how I felt about being "demoted" from being a senior NCO to second lieutenant, to which we both laughed. His last words as he shook my hand were, "Mike, I know you've given this community a lot, but we need you to come back to us as a doctor. I cannot tell you how valuable it will be to have a physician that has walked in your shoes and understands the mission. So, I hope you will consider giving the SOF community just a little bit more when the time comes." That was an easy ask, as it was exactly what I had intended all along.

"You can count on me, sir!" I replied as I saluted. He returned my salute with a smile and a punch in the upper arm before walking away.

All through medical school, when I heard people talking about choosing a specialty based on income or based on cushy lifestyle, all I was thinking about was how I could return to the SOF community and best support the mission. All I wanted was to get back to my tribe and to be around warriors again. It wasn't until after graduation, two years into my Emergency Medicine Residency, that I truly came to appreciate that not all doctors wearing a uniform thought as I did.

In medical residency training, a half day per week is set aside for educational lectures during what is known as "Grand Rounds." This is also true of medical residencies in the military, such as the one that I attended in San Antonio. One particular Grand Rounds lecture in my second year, an attending staff physician who had just returned from deployment to Iraq as an Infantry battalion surgeon was scheduled to speak for an hour on his experience in a theater of war. I was not alone among my classmates in eagerly anticipating this lecture, not only as a welcome respite from our typical boring didactics but also as a glimpse into what we could expect in just over a year, when we graduated and had the privilege to deploy ourselves. I was particularly excited because he was assigned to an *Infantry* battalion, as opposed to a support unit or a field hospital. While not special operations, an Infantry unit will always see its fair share of combat. I expected to hear a comprehensive overview of current trends in wound data, what equipment was being carried by medics and physicians, and any new innovations he had personally encountered and utilized in the realm of battlefield medicine. I was hoping for a "lessons learned" presentation that would give me a preview of what I could expect on deployment. Sadly, I was disappointed.

The ensuing PowerPoint presentation started with some pictures of his "pre-deployment training," which consisted of firing ranges and some basic soldier skills training. I was understanding of the fact that this was new and different to him, and many military physicians, so I wasn't at all put off by this. As the presentation continued, it seemed to more closely resemble someone showing pictures of their recent vacation as opposed to a summary of a combat tour: pictures of the plane ride over, with many smiling faces turning toward the camera; multiple angles of "my home away from home" showing his living space, complete with a bunk, a desk for his laptop, a TV, and an internet connection which he described as being "on the slow side but reliable." More pictures followed of aerial views of the Forward Operating Base (FOB) and the dining facility decked out in holiday splendor as he and his colleagues grinned widely over their cardboard trays of turkey and stuffing. After what seemed like forever, he finally put up a picture of his Battalion Aid Station (BAS), where he worked on a daily basis. I leaned forward in my chair, thinking we were getting to the real valuable stuff. He talked about the schedule that he had set up with his physician assistant and senior medic to see soldiers on "sick call" with minor complaints, such as sprains or runny noses, and talked about having his medics teach each other classes on various medical topics. There was no mention of treating combat trauma.

For a second, I thought I was the only one in the room that had noticed this omission, until one of my classmates raised their hand and specifically asked about treating trauma. The presenter stated that, because of their close proximity to a large theater-level field hospital, they did not see any trauma in his battalion aid station. He went on to say that he worked one night a week in that same field hospital's Emergency Department, but that he saw very few patients and used the time to "catch up on reading."

Just when I thought the presentation would be completely devoid of any useful information, the next slide showed the presenter dressed in full combat gear with a group of medics next to a Stryker armored vehicle with a red cross painted on the side and another photo showing the interior of the Stryker in its role as a Medical Evacuation Vehicle (MEV). He detailed how this vehicle would be dispatched with the Infantry vehicles to provide medical support on combat missions and that it would be crewed by three of his medics, or two medics and the battalion PA.

As he transitioned to the next slide and began talking about how he went about receiving "care packages" from his wife with some of his favorite snack foods and some much-needed power-converters, my hand shot up with the question that I felt was on everyone's mind. As soon as he looked in my direction, and before he even acknowledged my raised hand, I asked:

"Didn't you go out on missions? Did your battalion commander not allow it?"

The presenter chuckled and adjusted his glasses before answering.

"Really great question," he said. "When we arrived in theater, the surgeon from the battalion we replaced told me that he had been going out on missions both in the MEV and even on foot. After they left, I went to my commander and educated him on what a terrible idea that was. I explained that, for a board-certified EM physician to practice out in the field, without all of the interventions and tools that we are trained in, such as ultrasound, CAT scan, etc., it was the equivalent of putting an astronaut on a tricycle and expecting him to get to the moon."

"You see," he went on. "Sometimes one of your duties as battalion surgeon is to educate your commander on how to best utilize *you* as a resource. As an Infantry officer, he doesn't understand our level of education and that we aren't trained to practice medicine in the back of an armored vehicle or out of a backpack. He also might not understand that EM physicians are a valuable commodity to the Army and that we aren't as easy to replace as a medic or a PA. Great question! Thank you!"

I remember clenching my jaw and the sound of my own pulse in my ears as he continued with his slide show. I know he must have continued presenting for probably another 20 minutes. At some point, I just got up and walked out.

To me, it was incomprehensible that someone could be so blind and, in my opinion, cowardly. Allowing others with less training to bear the burden of treating wounded soldiers, while hiding behind weak excuses and surrounded by the safety of the FOB, was unthinkable to me. The entire reason I had gone to medical school in the first place was so that I could provide lifesaving care to those fighting *at the tip of the spear*. I was shocked and disgusted.

You may think that I am judging this physician too harshly, and you are entitled to that opinion. But the point I am making is that, even though he wore the uniform of a soldier, and even though he will carry the title "combat veteran" for the rest of his life, this man was not and will never be a warrior. A warrior would *never* choose the easy path. A warrior would *never* make excuses to stay behind. A warrior would *never* allow others to assume a risk that he would not assume himself. A warrior would put mission success above his personal safety. And, finally, a warrior would know in his heart that his rightful place is on the battlefield.

Ultimately, I came to realize that not everyone can lead a warrior lifestyle, and that's okay. The physician I described doesn't claim to be a warrior, and I don't begrudge his behavior on a personal level. It just runs contrary to my own ethos and how I have always chosen to live my life, both in and out of uniform.

In 2011, after serving three years in the JMAU, with two combat tours, two Bronze Star Medals (one with Valor), and receiving the Combat Medical Badge, I was given the chance to "hang up my spurs" and leave the unit honorably. At age 46, I could have coasted through the remaining time I had until my retirement and probably even avoided any further deployments. I chose not to. I chose to stay in the unit for an additional three years and to deploy three more times because that is what the mission required of me.

When I ultimately did retire, I could have taken a very lucrative job working ER shifts in a civilian hospital and left the warrior ethos behind. For a brief period, I tried that. My bank account was happy, but I was not. I also found myself having something of an identity crisis. It felt odd not identifying as a warrior any longer when I was still physically capable and mentally sharp. Knowing that I still had a lot more to give as a warrior, I chose to work fewer shifts for less money and dedicate more time to pursuits I felt to be more befitting of the warrior ethos.

I began working with both public and private organizations to teach combat trauma medicine to first responders and civilians. I volunteered to act as a medical director for law enforcement SWAT units. I increased the frequency and intensity of my training in martial arts and found work with companies teaching armed and unarmed defensive tactics. I started my podcast "Mind of The Warrior" as a means to share the ethos with others. And, of course, I launched the Greybeard Performance brand and wrote this book.

Throughout the course of this book I have discussed the ways that you can maximize both longevity and performance, how you should approach everything from sleep and nutrition to exercise and martial arts. Now, I want to discuss how to view that information through a warrior's eye.

PERFORMANCE VS. LONGEVITY

Whereas a soldier will follow orders and sacrifice longevity for performance when told to do so, a warrior recognizes that there is a balance between both. While a soldier might be nothing more than a chess piece to a commander, a warrior is a rare and valuable commodity. It is important that you embrace that balance and recognize that, as a warrior, you are needed not just for the battle at hand but for the entire war and for whatever future wars may come. A warrior also treats his body like the weapon that it is, which means caring for it in such a way that it will last for decades. It is said that the best thing an old warrior can teach a young warrior is how to become an old warrior, and to do that, you have to take care of yourself and continue to set an example.

AGING

In all warrior societies, the elders were respected and revered. To be an old warrior meant that you had been tested and survived what others could not. These "Greybeards" would mentor the younger warriors, who would recognize the value of their teachings. Older and more experienced warriors would progress in rank and would command others in combat. As they aged, they became more valuable for the depth of their knowledge as opposed to the swiftness of their sword. Aging warriors did not lament the fact that they could not throw a spear as far as they once had, nor that the weight of their shield now seemed heavier, but instead they celebrated the fact that they had survived numerous battles and that what they provided to the battle in their later years was even more valuable than what they provided in their youth. They knew their limitations and fully recognized how they could continue to be an asset and not a liability. There is a saying:

"The most common cause of injuries in old men is thinking that they are young men." Is it true? Probably not. But it illustrates a great point: you must have realistic expectations and use the wisdom of your experience to continue to be an asset as a warrior. King Leonidas of Sparta was 60 years old at the battle of Thermopylae, and you can bet that his men were extremely grateful to have his leadership and experience. It is doubtful (although not impossible) that he was ever in the front rank of the phalanx, but he was there, on the field of battle with his hoplon shield on his arm and a sharpened xiphos sword in his hand, and he led his men to the bitter end not only as a king, but as a *warrior*. Although your duties may be different, you can continue to be a warrior for as long as you draw breath on this earth.

SLEEP, DIET, AND NUTRITION

"An army marches on its stomach" is an old saying that still rings true. Whether we are talking about the Roman Legions of the Punic Wars, the Viking Hordes invading the British Isles, or the Allied Forces storming the beaches of Normandy on D-Day, the importance of keeping warriors properly fed cannot be overstated. In ancient times, the warriors always ate first and got the best food available. They recognized that over-indulging or eating the wrong foods could make them sluggish and ineffective in battle. When an army was on the march and made camp the night before battle, priority for a restful sleep went to those who would be at the tip of the spear in the morning, while those who would support them would stand watch and allow them to sleep. As a warrior lay in his tent, he would not let his mind dwell on the trivialities of daily life. Instead, he would calm himself and allow his body to sleep peacefully, knowing that he would need to be rested and alert for the coming battle. No battle has ever been won by lying awake and worrying about it the night before. Approach everything you put into your body as fuel for battle, and do not allow yourself to lay awake at night dwelling over past battles lost or worrying over the battles yet to come.

FITNESS AND RECOVERY

To say that physical fitness is extremely important in the life of a warrior would be a tremendous understatement. To lose a battle because your opponent is more skilled or has a superior battle plan is one thing, but to lose because of physical or mental exhaustion is never acceptable to a warrior. A warrior's priorities upon waking each morning are in assuring his weapons and equipment are ready for war, and this includes his body. A warrior will always make physical fitness a priority over leisure activities or pursuits of personal pleasure. This includes proper recovery, knowing that being physically fit makes little difference if you go into battle exhausted from yesterday's workout. On my deployments, I would work out first thing after waking every day, but I never exhausted myself to the point that I would be combat ineffective for the rest of the night (remember, we were always on reverse cycle). Once mission go/no-go decision was reached, if we did not have a mission for that night, I would do a second workout, knowing I could rest up before the next mission cycle. Never neglect your fitness and recovery. Never.

MARTIAL ARTS

To truly embrace the way of the warrior is to train in all forms of combat. I have met several high-level martial artists who have never spent a day in a military uniform but still live by the warrior ethos. Martial arts connect to the heart of the warrior in a way that is truly ancient. The practice of martial arts will help you cultivate the warrior mindset in a way that no other activity can, short of serving in actual combat. Even among active duty soldiers, including the Special Forces community, those who practice martial arts are a cut above their peers both physically and mentally. You see, being a warrior isn't simply about weapons proficiency, as I have seen "3 Gun" competitors who can shoot off a gnat's wings but who would be worthless in battle. It isn't simply about knowledge of tactics, as there are military historians who have memorized thousands of ancient battles in minute detail and yet couldn't plan an attack on the softest target imaginable. It isn't simply about physical fitness, or we would enlist all of our Olympic athletes and send them to war. Being a warrior is about mastery of self, and that is the heart of martial arts: self-mastery. Pursue martial arts, not just as a hobby, but as a way of life, and you will truly walk the path of a warrior.

SUPPLEMENTS AND HEALTH MAINTENANCE

Many natural and herbal supplements were discovered by warrior monks. Warriors of old knew when to seek a poultice or a salve, and they typically carried the makings of these in their kit while on the march. Warriors of ancient Egypt would chew on willow bark when they needed pain relief. This eventually led to the development of aspirin. During my time in the military, health maintenance was stressed in the form of regular physical exams and medical evaluations, particularly right before a deployment. Warriors know that the heat of battle is not the proper time to identify a hidden medical problem that could spell defeat. A warrior's body is his temple, and the temple must be maintained. Do not neglect your temple, and never allow yourself to become delinquent in the maintenance of your health.

YOUR TRIBE

In battle, you do not fight for flags or political ideals. You do not fight for lands or for glory. You fight for the warrior to your left and right, knowing that they will do the same for you. Those who have seen combat together share an unbreakable bond. In the words of the bard: "For whoever sheds his blood with me today shall be my brother." Although you may never enter into battle with your tribe, you will form a bond that is unique among warriors who live by the same ethos. As I said before, a tribe is about a shared philosophy and about accountability to one another. Find a tribe of like-minded warriors, and you will never have any doubt as to who will be there when you need them.

In closing, I hope that you have enjoyed this book and that you found at least some of it to be useful. Like anything, I encourage you to take what you like, leave what you don't, and improve upon it as you adapt it to your own life and lifestyle. You have a long way yet to go on this amazing journey that we call life, and every second is precious, so don't waste them by looking back on what "could have been" or the way it "used to be." You have no control over the days you have left behind; you only control those that stretch out in front of you, so make each day count, and relish every moment on this earth. Whatever life hands you, keep your head up, and keep bringing your best. Don't ever quit. Live life like a warrior.

Website: http://greybeardperformance.com

Instagram: @greybeardperformance

Facebook: https://www.facebook.com/GreybeardPerformance

ACKNOWLEDGMENTS

Writing this book would not have been possible without the help of some key individuals. My longtime friend and colleague Dr. Drew Winge, who was always there whenever I needed another set of eyes to help me validate the research on aging and supplements and introduced me to Brazilian Jiu Jitsu back when we were in residency. PJ Brownell, my fitness coach and friend, who helped me navigate the path to fitness as I reached my middle-50s and taught me that a rest day and a de-load is just as important as a challenging workout. My extended tribe, who continue to push me on the mats, in the gym, at the range, and in life, including all of the "Mind of The Warrior" listeners whose emails inspired me to keep podcasting and eventually write this book. Finally, to my brothers in arms who stood beside me. Whether it was in the steaming jungles of Colombia, in the scorched desert of Iraq, or on a frigid mountaintop in Afghanistan, those of us who made it through the fire to become the "Greybeards" have a duty to honor those who didn't make it home by sharing all that we have learned and by living each and every day to the fullest.

Rangers Lead The Way

De Oppresso Liber

Doc

Made in the USA
Coppell, TX
30 June 2022

79441063R00125